Asthma
Allergies
Children:
a parent's guide

PAUL EHRLICH, M.D.
LARRY CHIARAMONTE, M.D.
HENRY EHRLICH

3RD AVENUE BOOKS
BROOKLYN NY

While I am grateful to all those who have helped me in my medical career, I dedicate this book to my beloved wife Annemarie.

— *Dr. Larry Chiaramonte*

I would like to dedicate this book to my patients, who have taught me so much over so many years.

— *Dr. Paul Ehrlich*

Contents

Preface

THIS BOOK REPRESENTS HALF OF AN EXPERIMENT. IT IS BEING published in tandem with the launch of the website www.AsthmaAllergiesChildren.com. Our premise is that the science of allergies and asthma is constantly evolving, and that the web provides a medium for informing interested parties of new developments.

The website is aimed at two populations whose interests converge: parents of children who have allergies and asthma, and primary care physicians who are trying to treat them.

We have seen in decades of practice that parents of children with these conditions have a unique hunger for new information, and we offer the website as a town square for this community.

For their part, overworked general practitioners and pediatricians are providing more and more allergy and asthma treatment, and can benefit from regular access to specialists for the latest wisdom, or in many cases the *oldest* wisdom.

This peer-to-peer education is firmly in an old tradition. Practicing physicians have always learned from their colleagues who have been there and done that. The web affords us the chance to provide this kind of consultation at a distance.

The price of this book gives you entrée to this community. Parent or physician, now that you have bought the book, you are entitled to register at AsthmaAllergiesChildren.com and to participate in the give and take.

The book was originally published in 2002, which in Internet time is so last century. Not that the original isn't still valid—most of it is and has been retained. After all, as you will read, the human immune system has evolved over thousands of years, and our knowledge of how to treat it is progressing in fits and starts. At times we seem to be just treading water, and at others making dramatic breakthroughs.

What has changed is our ability to communicate about treatment. Let's start with the title of the first edition: *What Your Doctor May Not Tell You About Children's Allergies and Asthma: Simple Steps to Help Stop Attacks and Improve Your Child's Health.*

Whew. Doesn't exactly roll off the tongue, like *War and Peace*, or onto the browser either, for that matter. You put "asthma" and "allergies" into your search engine and it was a long time before you got to our book.

What else? The book was commissioned as part of a series that played on the idea that orthodox medicine deprived patients of knowledge, and that there were shortcuts to effective control. (One measure of the book's place in the media environment of our age: The original publisher was bought by a non-U.S. conglomerate, which pulled the plug on the whole series and the whole imprint.)

As you will read, there's nothing simple about allergies and asthma. Our methods are established science with a heavy dose of experience. For all that, we achieve good results—decades can go by between hospitalizations of our patients. Our patients live full lives, predominantly, and their parents are knowledgeable participants in treatment, but it can't be done with herbal tea and vitamins, not yet anyway. Effective treatment requires effort and adherence to proven means.

We now view the book as just one element of a communications strategy. Independent of any corporate marketing plan, our strategy is the result of almost eighty years with our allergic and asthmatic patients between us. The new book, with the functional, keyword-rich title *Asthma Allergies Children: A Parent's Guide*, is the mother ship, supported by AsthmaAllergiesChildren.com.

In the original book we noted that parents, patients and physicians are networked. Now we are building our own network. We were moved to take this step for several reasons. First, we can't republish the book every time there's a shift in medication, or in treatment protocols. For example, the last edition mentioned a medicine known as salmeterol, marketed as Serevent. Now, as you will read, use of salmeterol has been drastically curtailed because it was being used by some patients without an anti-inflammatory steroid, which posed a danger.

The web is a perfect vehicle for keeping our readers apprised of new developments, and we have linked to reputable organizations to make sure you have access to a full range of information.

Furthermore, we want to promote dialogue with our readers, both parents and doctors. As we say in chapter 14, informed parents teach one another in ways that doctors can't always do, but the best support groups are affiliated with doctors who ensure the soundness of information. We propose to take that role here. We want parents to take what they learn here to their own family physicians, particularly primary care doctors who will continue to do the lion's share of treatment, and we want those doctors to communicate with us.

As of this writing, health care reform legislation has finally been passed and signed into law. We hope that the provisions dedicated to evidence-based medicine and best practices will make health care both more effective and economical. It is worth noting that Dr. Atul Gawande of Harvard, writing about the law's implementation the week after it was signed (*New Yorker*, April 5, 2010), told of a program at Boston Children's Hospital that takes a systematic, preventive approach for inner-city children that parallels work both of us have done in New York. In Boston, insurance pays for inhalers, while the hospital carries the costs of nurses who visit parents after discharge, enforcing compliance with medication and home hygiene. "After a year," Dr. Gawande writes, "the hospital readmission rate for these patients dropped by more than eighty per cent, and costs plunged. But an empty hospital bed is a revenue loss, and asthma is Children's Hospital's leading source of admissions. Under the current system, this sensible program could threaten to bankrupt it."

The 80 percent reduction in emergency treatment is almost exactly what allergy specialists have been reporting for a generation, but sadly, this also reveals how our medical economy has come to depend on ineffective treatment.

We anticipate that under the Patient Protection and Affordable Care Act, the lessons of Boston Children's will be remembered as change works its way through the system as a whole. It is patients, not institutions, that count. But we are not waiting for full implementation of reform. We have written this book and the website to put information in the hands of parents and family physicians and help achieve what Boston Children's did, one family or one family *practice*, at a time.

We are both senior physicians. That means we are old. But we hope that age and experience have given us wisdom that will benefit you the reader. And age hasn't stopped us from learning. As you will read, both of us have devoted a considerable amount of time to bringing the best of allergy and immunology to underserved, high-risk populations, which has given us new insight into how chronic disease can be managed. Still, we have learned over many years that a child doesn't have to be poor to have his life drastically diminished by asthma and allergies. We want to reach them all.

Asthma
Allergies
Children:
a parent's guide

CHAPTER 1

Introduction to Allergy

IF YOU ARE THE PARENT OF AN ALLERGIC CHILD, YOU VERY LIKELY suffer from allergies yourself. You know the misery allergies can bring, on a scale from annoying itching of skin and eyes at one end, to debilitating sneezing fits in the middle, to life-threatening asthma attacks or anaphylactic shock at the other. You know how allergies can be misdiagnosed. You know about drowsiness induced by some antihistamines, and the inconvenience of carrying nebulizers and inhalers. You know how the joy of childhood can be diminished by eternal vigilance about foods, activities, and environments.

We know about them, too. We are both board-certified pediatric allergists. For some sixty years between the two of us, we have been treating children like yours, and from what we have seen, the prognosis for allergy treatment is troubling.

For one thing, allergies seem to be becoming more common.

Part of this is due to changes in the way we live. We live in homes that are sealed to trap heat in the winter and cool conditioned air in the summer. We have wall-to-wall carpeting and throw rugs on our floors. But this comfortable and energy-conscious approach creates an environment in which dust mites thrive. Energy efficiency means that there is less fresh air from outside being exchanged with stale air indoors, which means that dust builds up inside. Carpeting may be comfortable to walk on, insulating, and attractive, but stuff that settles in it is fodder for dust mites, and their waste is highly allergenic.

In a sense, allergy is a price we have paid for progress. Part of the body's defenses, the immune system, evolved to help us fight off parasites when our ancestors had very little ability to influence either their environment or their diet. Now that we do have such power, that mechanism has gone haywire. The first great impetus for the development of allergies may have been the invention of shoes, which kept worms or other parasites from entering our feet and thereby put parts of the immune system out of work. Frank T. Vertosick, Jr., author of a book called *The Genius*

Within: Discovering the Intelligence of Every Living Thing, advances the theory that the brain is not the only part of the body that can learn from experience. He writes, "The immune system must learn and recall billions, perhaps trillions, of different molecular patterns. Our lives depend on its ability to make instant discriminations between friend and foe, not an easy task." While our specialty is Allergy and Immunology, we will reserve judgment on whether this constitutes "intelligence" or not. However, we never cease to wonder at the resourcefulness of the immune system, not only its resiliency in combating disease, but also its potential for mischief when it goes awry.

Because of modern sanitation, climate control, and immunization, many of the original problems the immune system evolved to combat no longer exist routinely in advanced industrial countries like ours. However, the defenses are still within us. Like soldiers demobilized at the end of a war, they need time to adjust after the fighting stops, but in the case of immunity that has evolved over eons, the adjustment hasn't begun. Idle hands make the devil's work. These are defenses in search of an enemy, and they spend their time attacking all kinds of things—molds, pollens, chemicals used in the construction of our homes—and in the process of attacking those irritants, they throw off toxins that make us sick.

There's a saying that what children need in their homes to keep allergies from developing is a pound of dirt, as would be the case on a farm. That theory recently gained support in a study published in the *New England Journal of Medicine* (Sept. 19, 2002) saying that infants raised in homes with two or more cats and dogs developed allergies at roughly half the rate as children in pet-free homes. Moreover, they were less allergic not just to dogs and cats but to pollens and other common allergens as well. Other studies have supported those findings, but others have not, and we remain equivocal, as we were in 2002.

The newest wrinkle is experimentation with hookworms, which are common in regions where people defecate in outdoor latrines and come into contact with their waste by walking barefoot in the designated areas. Epidemiologists have established that where hookworms are prevalent, allergies and asthma are unknown, possibly because they keep an antibody called IgE busy doing something constructive instead of attacking harmless proteins, which is the basis of allergic disease. You will read more about this in these pages.

While we would like to see natural processes harnessed to fight allergy, however, this throwback science is not proven, whereas the incidence of pernicious anemia and other conditions associated with hookworm are quite well known. Research is ongoing, particularly at the University of Nottingham in England.

Still, it is legitimate to ask, if progress is causing all that trouble, if our environment is too antiseptic, is worth it? Or should we just move into mud huts with no indoor toilets? We'll leave that to philosophers. In the meantime, we have the obligation to try to keep ahead of our bodies' own defenses. Science allows us to give it a try. And what the science says is that the jury is still out on exposing children to cats and dogs to try to protect them against allergies, as the authors of the study were among the first to point out. After all, the data cited in the study were contrary to long-established wisdom and practice on the subject. It may well be a statistical anomaly. The results must be repeatable. So, much to the consternation of animal-loving new parents in families with a history of allergy, we must advise that they *not* run out to the animal shelter and stock up on new pets.

Why Treatment May Be Getting Worse

The science is good, and it's getting better. As the understanding of allergy grows, so does the effectiveness of drugs to treat various conditions, as well as environmental adjustments to minimize attacks. Still, treatment may be getting worse.

And it's not for want of effort. Many general practitioners and family practitioners are doing more to treat allergy than their counterparts did when we began practice decades ago. Indeed, a generation ago, most GPs (general practitioners) and pediatricians didn't even acknowledge allergy as something to be taken very seriously. One of your authors—Dr. Ehrlich—is the son of a late and much respected pediatrician who rarely referred any of his patients to allergists, even when his own son became one. Instead, children and their parents were given antihistamines and counseled to put up with sneezing. Skin conditions were treated with all-purpose ointments and creams. Bad asthma attacks were controlled with systemic cortisone, which would affect the whole body, not just the lungs. Prolonged cortisone use had substantial long-term side effects.

Today, we know what works to keep asthma under control, but doctors don't always do it. In 1990 and 1991 the National Institutes of Health (NIH) convened experts under the leadership of Albert Sheffer, MD, from Harvard Medical School to produce guidelines for the treatment of this growing threat to public health. However, as the *Journal of Asthma* has pointed out, more than a decade later, these treatment guidelines are not followed in 50 percent of cases, although as the most recent NIH data show, treatment has never been safer or more effective. (The American Academy of Allergy, Asthma & Immunology has position statements on treatments currently deemed effective at www.aaaai.org.)

The largest and most comprehensive study of the quality of children's health care in the U.S. reached disquieting conclusions, as reported in the *New England Journal of Medicine* (Oct. 11, 2007). While children received the appropriate treatment for acute conditions like colds 92 percent of the time, children with asthma got the appropriate care just 46 percent of the time—exactly half as frequently. This means that more often than not, they were deprived of appropriate care. Inadequately treated asthmatic children are more likely to fail at school, more likely to lose out on sports and other activities, more likely to miss out on the fun and challenges of childhood, and more likely to be less productive as adults.

While part of the needlessly high incidence of asthma is the fault of doctors, there's also blame to be found in the behavior of patients, and patients' parents. The parents have misgivings about a diagnosis of asthma, so their doctor will treat their child for "bronchitis" instead. They don't want their child to take corticosteroids because they confuse them with the drugs that athletes take. They don't want to pay $20 out of pocket for a peak flow meter because their insurance won't pay for it. They want fast-acting relief drugs, not controller drugs that must be taken even when they don't have symptoms. These treatments are all part of the NIH guidelines, yet they are commonly overlooked. Some 70 percent of asthma patients never refill their control medication, which is one reason we have 2 million emergencies due to asthma.

Referrals to Allergists—Still Dwindling

Despite all we know about effective treatment, referrals to allergists are dwindling. Part of the trouble is that allergy is still not taken seriously even at some of the best teaching hospitals. New York University, where Dr. Ehrlich studied, is just one of the major teaching hospitals that offer no training in allergy. He gained his certification on a postgraduate fellowship while serving in the U.S. Navy. When you consider the concentration of graduates of teaching hospitals in the New York metropolitan area, and that New York is to medical training roughly what Vermont is to maple syrup, you can see the structural difficulties to getting more explicit recognition of allergy as a specialty.

The same holds true elsewhere in the country. The division on allergy treatment is clearly delineated by attitudes at the different medical schools. It should surprise no one that the people who work at medical schools with no allergy program tend to feel that they have enough allergists, while those that have a program want more. The attitudes fall under the heading of whether the glass is half empty or half full. Schools that are not allergy-oriented feel it is enough for general practitioners to treat allergy with medication. Allergy-oriented schools view this treatment as superficial, and believe in full investigation and treatment with allergen avoidance in the diet and environment, building up the body's own resistance through immunotherapy (see chapter 9), and behavioral change.

The problem is compounded by ripple effects. We live in a networked society. Doctors' referrals are determined by their connections through medical school, internship, residency, hospital affiliation, and so on—and can be limited to specialists who take one kind of insurance or another. If a doctor is networked to institutions that don't treat allergy properly, his patients are going to miss out.

Finally, there is the problem of the way we pay for treatment.

Insurance companies often make it more profitable for primary care physicians to care for patients' allergies themselves instead of referring them to allergists. The primary care doctor may be directly rewarded if he doesn't make a specialty referral. He may also choose to perform a broad battery of tests because he gets paid for each. An allergist, on the other hand, may be able to rule out some possible allergens without testing. Furthermore, some tests,

5

as you will read in chapter 7, may provide misleading information and overtreatment. This can be especially problematic in the case of food allergy, as you will read in chapter 5. Patients pay the price in time lost from school and work, in poorer long-term health, in expensive emergency care, and, not infrequently, malnutrition. The direct costs of medical care for asthma alone, including doctors' visits, hospitalization, drugs, and so on, along with indirect costs such as absences from work or school, are billions of dollars a year. In 2005 one of your authors, Dr. Ehrlich, created Project E.R.A.S.E (Eradicating Respiratory Asthma in Schools to help children Excel), which sends specialists into high-need inner-city schools. In the first year, hospitalizations fell from twenty-six to six, saving about $125,000 in medical costs. These children had previously been treated only by pediatricians, general practitioners, and emergency room physicians.

General Care Versus Specialist Care and Your Child

How does this shift from allergy care to primary care affect you and your child? While both doctors will pick from the same pool of allergy and asthma medication, the allergist has more experience using it. The allergist will pick those that are easier to use and will more likely use preventive medication, teaching both patient and parent how to adjust the dosage to symptoms. He will investigate the source of the allergies and teach you how to reduce your child's exposure. He may have access to very modern technology that can precisely measure lung inflammation and prescribe precisely calibrated dosages. When indicated, he will start immunotherapy and will draw on his experience to give the proper dose for safety and benefit. Finally, he will reinforce the behavioral changes needed to keep the condition from reaching a crisis point. This all takes time, and the point is that the allergist will take the time, while a GP may not.

Shrinking Ranks

The long-term trends about the medical specialty of allergy are disturbing. When you consider that 15 to 20 percent of Americans currently suffer from allergies of some kind, including 35 million from allergic rhinitis, that 15 million have asthma, that 2 percent suffer from food allergies including 6 to 8 percent of children, and that the numbers in all categories are increasing, you might think that demand for specialist care would also be increasing too. Yet for all the advances, the pool of allergy specialists is shrinking. There are fewer board-certified allergists than there were ten years ago. Fewer, in fact, than any specialty except for rectal surgeons, and the pool of allergists is getting older.

In 2001, the year before we wrote the first version of this book, eighty fewer board-eligible doctors finished allergy residency programs than the year before, which is consistent with a long-standing trend. The percentage of graduates from good programs like those at Johns Hopkins, Einstein, Yale and Harvard who were choosing research instead of actually treating patients was increasing, which boded well for the basic science, but not the delivery of treatment. In any case, the potential pool of new practicing allergists is still diminishing, even as the number of current practitioners is shrinking due to retirement. There are only 5,000–6,000 board-certified allergists out of 600,000 practicing MDs in the United States, and as of late 2009, just over 300 doctors were in accredited training programs for allergy and immunology, compared to more than 22,000 for internal medicine. Since allergy programs are at least two years, roughly 150 new allergists are produced each year. (Figures are from the Accreditation Council for Graduate Medical Education.) If allergists have a thirty-year career, then some 170–200 retire each year, for a net loss in the pool of board-certified allergists. The problem is complicated further by the fact that many of those residents will go into research, not into clinical practice at the same time many allergists are getting older. There's no way to measure exactly how many of our colleagues are retiring, but when we go to conferences, there are more doctors who look the way we do now than there were thirty-five years ago.

The Overworked GP

It's not the GP's fault. An article in the *American Journal of Public Health* in April 2003 pointed to an acute medical problem—a lack of time. As reported in the *New York Times*, the study says that if GPs follow the *existing* preventive protocols recommended by the federal government for just thirty common medical issues, including "tests for breast and colon cancer, high blood pressure and high cholesterol, as well as counseling on alcohol and tobacco use, exercise and seat belt use," they would have no time left in a seven-hour day to actually treat anyone.

The problem has grown because of the way doctors have been compensated. Dr. Lisa Sanders of Yale and Waterbury Hospital in Connecticut, who wrote the wonderful book *Every Patient Tells a Story*, says, "Doctors are paid to do, not to think." That is, giving shots and doing tests pay better than long thoughtful conversations about a patient's life, which, as you will see, is the kind of medicine that an allergist practices.

Overworked GPs, pediatricians, and others who serve as primary care physicians (PCPs) shouldn't have to see patients every eleven minutes to make an honest living, and then spend two hours a night answering phone calls and doing paperwork. Recently enacted health care reform will not change this any time soon. It remains to be seen how that will change, if it will change, or indeed, whether any reform will ensure that adequate numbers of PCPs can give every patient a so-called medical home with access to specialty allergy care.

Then there's the problem of continuing education. They are dealing with a moving target, and it's hard to keep up.

Consider that in the two major conferences and the two leading professional journals dedicated to allergy there are some 2,000 articles published or presented every year that are peer-reviewed, meaning they have been read by scientists for importance and accuracy. That is just the tip of the iceberg when you take into account all the research that is going on, with sponsorship by pharmaceutical companies, foundations, and universities. That's a lot for a busy GP. And when you add the reading in ophthalmology, neurology, gastroenterology, pulmonology, infectious disease, and cardiology, you can appreciate the burden of remaining current.

Moreover, there's an allergy component to many other specialties that should be understood, starting with prenatal diet. For example, women with a propensity to allergy should avoid eggs, milk, peanuts, and other high-allergy foods during their third trimester of pregnancy and while breast-feeding, in order to minimize the chances that the

---

THE ALLERGIST DIFFERENCE

Carole was a 7-month-old infant whose 32-year-old mother had herself long put up with allergic rhinitis and the stuffed nose and sneezing that accompanies it in springtime. Carole did well, breast-feeding exclusively, until 4 months of age when, soon after the introduction of solids, she began to develop eczema. She started snorting and developed nasal congestion. Changing foods helped only slightly, and Mother sought the help of a pediatric allergist. A review of which foods had caused the initial problem revealed a possible problem with wheat cereal. It was discontinued. However, a more careful history revealed that Mother was fond of wheat and made it a large part of her own diet. Because Mother was continuing breast-feeding, the allergist suggested stopping all wheat in *her* diet as well.

Subsequently, Carole's symptoms went away, and she is now being followed for additional nonfood allergies. It is important to establish in every instance how allergens enter the body.   — *Dr. Chiaramonte*

---

allergy clock will start running early for their allergy-prone offspring. Once that clock does start ticking, it's fairly predictable and difficult for both child and parent. Painful conditions like colic, vomiting, and general crankiness, which take a toll on parental nerves in addition to children's health, can be followed by eczema and other symptoms.

The conventional wisdom is that the child will probably outgrow one problem or another. They might, but chances are that each condition they outgrow will be followed by another down the road—accompanied by the psychological problems that come from having spent their childhood sneezing, wheezing, and scratching.

Without ready access to input from allergists, our overworked GPs and internists will treat allergies either in isolation, or in the context of other ostensibly more serious conditions. They will ignore the connection between allergies and asthma, when in fact they are linked to one another. Unable to recognize the specifics of a particular condition, they take an overly broad approach in testing and then prescribe medications that are at the trailing edge of treatment for a particular condition when a leading-edge treatment exists. Or they will prescribe a treatment that has a much smaller efficacy rate than others that are available. The result is comparable to what happens when a writer uses a thesaurus without using a dictionary. Two words may be synonyms on the surface, but when the wrong one is used in a sentence, the result may be highly misleading.

Long-Term Damage When Allergy Slips Through the Cracks

In one emergency department in New York City that is supervised by a colleague of ours, approximately one-third of the children treated for acute asthma are not previously known to have had asthma and had never been treated for it. This could be because the child had never had a previous asthma attack, or such an attack went undiagnosed or was treated as a different type of medical disorder. Moreover, as you will read in chapter 8, "The Hows and Whys of Allergy and Asthma Medication," both patients and their family physicians tend to concentrate on short-term relief rather than ongoing disease control. Regardless, there is a great amount of denial on the part of both patient and parents where asthma is concerned. They simply don't want to believe asthma is present, or that it is an ongoing condition in the absence of overt symptoms.

This can be disastrous in the long run. We have learned that asthma is a cumulative condition. The lungs may be permanently weakened not only by each attack but also by the presence of non-symptomatic asthma—asthma that produces no overt symptoms but results in damage from underlying inflammation. Prolonged trial and error in finding the right treatment and intermittent use of medication are things your child cannot afford.

Moreover, even if GPs were capable of providing equivalent treatment, the sheer economics of general practice wouldn't allow it. GPs screen hundreds of conditions. Anyone who has sat in the waiting room of a family practitioner or a pediatrician knows that you almost never get to see a doctor without waiting at least an hour after the appointment time. Allergy diagnosis and treatment literally take more time than the GP can spare. It's hard to devote the time it takes to consider the particulars of a child's condition when the economics of practice are based on the three minutes it takes to diagnose an ear infection and write a prescription. And once you get to see the doctor, he may treat the symptoms instead of the underlying problem. Alleviating symptoms is important to stave off cumulative damage, but hyposensitization to allergenic agents through a course of immunotherapy demands an intricate course of testing and treatment with detailed adjustment for the best dosage.

You wouldn't want your mechanic to replace your brakes every time you hear a squeak—a small adjustment might work. At the same time, you would want him to tell you that if you change your driving habits, you might save a lot of wear and tear. As Dr. Mark Ballow, president of the American Academy of Allergy, Asthma & Immunology puts it, "Any doctor can prescribe Advair [a control medication]. An allergist can reduce the need for it."

Imprecise treatment takes a toll on individual patients, on their families and on the health care system as a whole, including taxpayers and all those who have to pay for their own health insurance. A single hospitalization for asthma costs taxpayers or insurers more than clinical treatment by a board-certified allergist for a year.

Is specialist care effective? For a start, neither one of us has had a patient in more than a decade who required hospitalization due to asthma. The fact that allergy care *can* be treated in a GP's office doesn't mean that it *should* be. It's a misallocation of valuable time. Working with specialists makes GPs better doctors. There shouldn't be a tug-of-war over the treatment dollar. We're partners in patient treatment. We help each other do the best for the patient.

Better Living Through Better Living

Fifty years ago, a major chemical company used the slogan "Better Living Through Chemistry" to describe its work in making things like synthetic fibers and fertilizers. That was at the height of post–World War II faith in technology. Since then we have all learned that many technologies have their shortcomings and unwanted side effects. Certainly chemistry plays a pivotal role in controlling your child's allergies, but it doesn't do everything, and it can't. To a great extent, we have to give the body a chance to do some of the work for us, and to a further extent, we have to control the damage by not provoking our children's immune systems to work against them in the first place. As you will see, we are great believers in immunotherapy and in altering behavior to keep bad things from happening.

Networked Patients

We remarked earlier that the medical professionals in your life are networked, and that the weaknesses in allergy treatment in one medical practice are very likely shared throughout the doctor's network of hospital affiliations, specialist alliances and, above all, insurance plans.

Patients and parents of patients like yourselves, however, are largely on your own. This book is for you. We don't believe that you should use it to become an expert on the subject of allergy and asthma treatment, but rather to become a more educated, discerning, demanding patient or parent of a patient.

There are networks of people communicating through websites, some good, some bad. We talk with many support groups and indeed run meetings in our own offices. We recommend that you join a support group because it can be a cost-efficient way to educate yourself about the full panoply of medication and behavioral change necessary to effectively control a condition. And because people in such groups have already translated technical information into lay terminology, they can be better at explaining and reinforcing information than doctors alone, with our Babel of Greek, Latin, and medical jargon.

But a word of caution here: Because the science of allergy is very involved and rapidly developing, and because commonly available medical treatment can fall wide of the mark, patients and patients' parents in their frustration are susceptible to misleading or false advice. Poorly supervised support groups are greenhouses for quack solutions and they grow like weeds. How can you tell a good group from a bad group? Talk about it with your specialist. But as a rule of thumb, avoid recommendations that endorse a magic bullet solution, that leave out hard science, that overemphasize certain foods, or that depend on tests chosen according to what your insurance will pay for.

We have a good deal more to say about these and other topics in the pages that follow. We hope that by the time you have finished reading you will find, as our thousands of patients have over many years, that allergies are annoying and require care, but that they don't have to be debilitating or dangerous.

A Network of Our Own

The Internet has revolutionized communications. With the publication of this edition, we are embarking on some networking of our own by creating www.AsthmaAllergiesChildren.com, the complementary website we mentioned in the preface. We will use it to update users with the latest in the literature, and allergy- and asthma-related news. Each person who buys this book can be part of our community and participate in our blog and other interactive capabilities as we add them. When you visit AsthmaAllergiesChildren.com, you will see a parents' inbox and a physicians' inbox. In each we will receive queries from and provide answers to the pertinent group. The physician outreach is especially dear to our hearts because we want to extend our knowledge to a wider population of physicians. The fact is that there's no doctor worth his or her degree who hasn't benefited as much from consulting colleagues as they have from years of training and residency. Each of us has learned in this way. And we would like to provide the same courtesy to our colleagues in primary practice. Together, in this triangular setting—parents on one corner, primary care physicians on another, and ourselves on the third—we can make a real difference in the lives of all those beloved little patients out there.

When Cells Attack:
The Mechanics of Allergy

A S WE SAID IN CHAPTER 1, ALLERGIES ARE ESSENTIALLY DEFENSES against parasites looking for something to do when there are no more parasites. On one level, you can think of them as guard dogs suddenly turned loose into neighborhoods to fend for themselves with no retraining after they are no longer needed for guard duty. Anything that moved would be in grave danger.

But if that were the only problem, we could deal with it. In fact, the danger is even more insidious because it's not just a question of swarming dog packs being rounded up again. There are not only immediate effects of allergic reaction, but also secondary ones that have only been treatable for a few years and tertiary ones that we're just learning about that may be the most dangerous of all.

In this chapter, we are going to discuss how allergy works because understanding the allergy process will help give you a feel for what is going on in your child's body, make you a more knowledgeable partner with your physicians in treatment, and give you a sense of urgency about why it is so important to help your child follow your allergist's treatment program, as well as follow his or her suggestions about controlling the home environment.

Altered State

The word allergy comes from the Greek *allos*, which literally means "altered state." The body has the ability to recognize something foreign. Your body can distinguish something that belongs to itself from something that does not. It reacts to the foreign substance in a specific way largely by producing antibodies or immunoglobulins that wrap around the foreign substances the way a glove does around a hand; to paraphrase the late Johnnie Cochrane, if the antibodies fit, they must attack it. The pertinent antibodies for allergic response are called IgE antibodies, as we mentioned in chapter 1. What's more, the immune system has a memory. Each time it is exposed to the same foreign material, more antibodies are produced, faster than before. This is called the amnestic, or memory, response. Each time antibodies encounter the antigens they are made to fight, a chain reaction begins. Each antibody type can start different chain reactions, some of which are merely uncomfortable and some of which are dangerous.

In one sense, everyone is allergic. The ability to distinguish things that belong in your body from those that don't is the basis of the entire immune system, even for those who don't have allergies as we are using the term. We may remember from high school science classes about all those phagocytes and other killer cells attacking infection. That's the benign side of the immune system: It's life-saving and necessary. When an infectious agent—virus or bacteria—is detected, the immune system responds by sending out antibodies that seek to contain and kill it. You can think of it as a police action. The police respond to a report of a burglary and go arrest the perpetrator. Afterward, the victim wires his home with an alarm system linked to the police station and thereby immunizes his home against further crime, he hopes.

Jump-Starting the Immune System

We jump-start the immune systems of our children by vaccinating them against common diseases such as rubella and diphtheria, which saves the lives and health of millions of children but has become controversial because certain difficult-to-explain phenomena such as autism or the occurrence of severe brain damage are sometimes attributed to them.

Originally, vaccination took place naturally through exposure to certain germs. If you studied the history of smallpox in biology, you will recall that the effective elimination of this deadly disease began when scientist Edward Jenner learned that by exposing people to a weak virus called cowpox, which was found on dairy farms, the body would produce immunity to the virulent smallpox as well. People who worked with cows enjoyed this immunity without medical intervention. By encountering cowpox while milking cows, their bodies were prompted to make antibodies specific for killing the invading bacteria.

The trick—and it's a big one—is to find a vaccine that provokes the production of antibodies without causing the disease. The original polio vaccine developed by Jonas Salk did this by using dead polio virus, but it was only partially effective and needed to be administered repeatedly. The more potent vaccine, created by Albert Sabin, used a live virus that had certain disease-producing components removed.

Like the spontaneously produced antibodies that cause natural immunity, all vaccines are specific to particular diseases. When the two of us were younger, universal smallpox vaccine effectively wiped out the plague of smallpox as it existed in nature, and the ability to recognize and fight smallpox bacteria faded. When this happens, we need "booster shots" to refresh the production of new antibodies. This is noteworthy now because the threat of bioterrorism has revived smallpox vaccination.

Immune Systems Gone Wild

Sometimes the immune system breaks down. Press coverage of the AIDS epidemic told us that HIV (human immunodeficiency virus) gradually exhausts the body's ability to combat the virus. Killer T cells attack HIV but the virus is resourceful and regenerates itself in new variations that find ways of circumventing medication. This literally wears out the immune system. Deprived of their defenses, most AIDS patients die from "opportunistic infections"—illnesses such as pneumonia that someone with a fully functioning immune system would be able to fight off. This is the physiological equivalent of the collapse of the Soviet Union. A fragile economic system was toppled by the chronic burdens of fighting a war in Afghanistan and trying to match the United States in nuclear weaponry. Even healthy economies can collapse if they have to fight wars all the time.

Another newsworthy discussion of the immune system comes from advances in organ transplant technology. People who receive a new heart or liver face a lifetime of medication to keep their bodies from rejecting the new organ. The body is effectively "allergic" to the new organ, much as we would like it not to be.

Occasionally the immune system goes completely haywire. The diseases rheumatoid arthritis and lupus are the body's equivalent of a police state: The immune system attacks healthy tissue in the joints and organs. Chronic inflammation can be progressively disfiguring, crippling, and deadly.

Destructive Functioning of Normal Systems

The complexity of allergy stems from the complexity of the immune system itself. The immune system is not one thing but is really a group of interlocking subsystems that utilize some of their beneficial functions in a harmful fashion. When we use the word "allergy" we really mean the normal functioning of the immune system in these destructive ways.

Three Reactions to Antigens

When the body initially encounters an allergen—what's known as *primary exposure*—it can react in one of three ways, two of which are positive or harmless and the third of which is allergic.

The first is *immunization*: The body produces normal antibodies that will attack the allergen and kill it through a sequence of activity by T cells and B cells. Antibodies are also called *immunoglobulins*. The most important beneficial one is called immunoglobulin G, or IgG.

The second is *tolerance*: There will be no immune response at all because the body can simply coexist with the substance, a kind of physiological "don't ask, don't tell" policy.

Third is *sensitization*: This results from the production of the antibody IgE, which then attaches itself to the receptors on two kinds of cells, *mast cells*, and *basophils* (although there may be others as well). However these cells, particularly the mast cell, are most important for our purposes here because their action produces most of the problems related to allergy. Each antibody is dedicated to fighting a single allergen—really just a few proteins in those allergens. People with multiple allergies have a variety of IgE cells attached to the mast cells programmed to different allergens. As you can see, with all those antibodies floating about, treating multiple allergies can be a tricky business.

The mast cell was discovered by Dr. Paul Ehrlich (no relation to the co-author), who was most famous for his development of "Dr. Ehrlich's magic bullet," the first effective treatment for syphilis. Mast cells are nature's command center and arsenal rolled into one. But they are remarkably undiscriminating. Do you know the expression "If you're a hammer, everything looks like a nail"? To a mast cell, every time an allergen appears for which it has a specific IgE antibody, that allergen looks like a life-threatening parasite.

The mast cell is present in all tissue in greater or lesser concentrations. Upon initial exposure to an allergen, or antigen (remember that you don't become allergic the first time you encounter these substances), antibodies attach themselves by the thousands to the receptors of the mast cell.

The "claws" of the IgE antibodies stick out, and work in pairs. They look something like lobster claws. The allergens fit between the "claws," forming a bridge, and when they do, the allergic attack begins. The mast cell swells up and bursts and *mediators* are released.

After a mast cell does its work, it looks like a piñata after children have pounded it with sticks and all the toys and candy have been unwrapped. Without medical intervention, the mast cell uses all the weapons in its arsenal, and alerts other cells, such as *eosinophils*, to show up and do their work. It's as if a home burglar alarm went off and the police responded without stopping to figure out whether the cat tripped the alarm or Public Enemy Number One was holed up inside. The police might show up and burst in the front door, or they might break it down, or they might enter with tear gas and guns blazing.

The allergy equivalents might be sneezing or itching in one case, hives or wheezing in another, or life-threatening *anaphylactic shock* in another. One child's healthy school lunch can send another to the hospital. This range of symptoms and reactions is what makes the process of diagnosis and treatment so difficult for the nonspecialist.

An Allergy Attack, Step by Step

What happens when your daughter gets hay fever? Ragweed pollen lodges in her nose. If she didn't have hay fever, it would just be treated like any other kind of dirt and make its way back through the sinuses into the throat where it would be swallowed, and eventually destroyed by stomach acid.

But because she has an allergy, she is about to embark on an episode of allergic rhinitis. Mast cells start gathering in the nasal passages to attack the intruder. The IgE receptors adhering to the outside of the

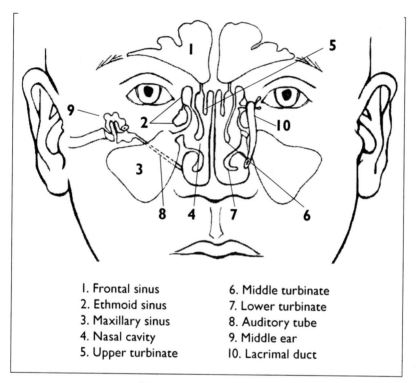

1. Frontal sinus
2. Ethmoid sinus
3. Maxillary sinus
4. Nasal cavity
5. Upper turbinate

6. Middle turbinate
7. Lower turbinate
8. Auditory tube
9. Middle ear
10. Lacrimal duct

Figure 1. Normal sinuses

mast cells attach themselves to the allergen. As more and more of these cells are delivered by the blood as it circulates, serum or plasma—the liquid part of the blood—starts to accumulate. Once activated, the mast cells start to *degranulate*, releasing mediators—primarily histamine—which go to work destroying the allergen.

The allergy attack progresses from an itching sensation and runny nose to an overwhelming urge to expel the intruder physically, known in common parlance as a sneeze, to production of stronger mediators and initiation of even stronger protective measures, including the production of mucus, which coats and then clogs the sinuses. The tissue becomes engorged and inflamed. The sneezing stops, but nothing can get in or out of your child's nose, and she starts to breathe through her mouth. This progression of symptoms and responses is basically the same for every allergic attack, although the amount of damage eventually done varies according to where symptoms are felt and the severity of the allergies.

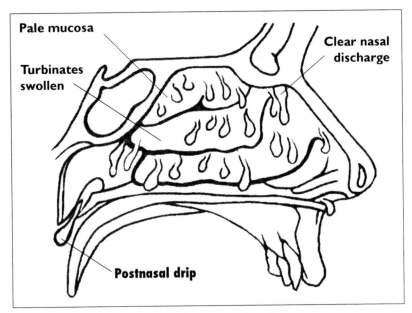

Pale mucosa

Clear nasal discharge

Turbinates swollen

Postnasal drip

Figure 2. Allergic rhinitis
What's green and goes backwards?
Those mucous membranes are kicking into overdrive—the dripping
starts, the tissues swell up, and your child is miserable.

First Level of Allergy

For many years, medical science was directed at acute allergic symptoms such as runny nose from pollens, say, or itchy eyes from exposure to cats, or angry swelling from a mosquito bite. In most cases, the symptoms would subside in a few hours although attacks such as bee stings might be deadly to certain people. These temporary symptoms were all in response to a single mediator, *histamine*.

Histamine is nature's equivalent of an over-the-counter remedy to the perceived attack. It is contained, ready-mixed, in the mast cells, which are, as mentioned above, circulating in the blood at all times, ready to gravitate toward the site of exposure to an allergen, such as the skin, the respiratory system, the gastrointestinal tract, and the eyes.

Since the allergic response is outwardly a matter of discomfort that will eventually subside, the first line of defense has been to use an *antihistamine*. More serious reactions were for many years attributed to a secondary mediator, what was referred to as slow-reacting substances of anaphylaxis (SRS-A), produced in quantities sufficient to cause anaphylactic shock, and requiring emergency treatment. As you will see, this was a simplistic view of what was really going on. We now know that histamine not only fights the allergen itself but triggers a chain reaction of other cellular responses that last for hours and can cause long-term discomfort or cumulative damage. The secondary agents are not just a single substance, SRS-A, but a much more complex set of ingredients.

Histamine is a fascinating substance. It lurks in the mast cells, ready to do duty attacking intruders. It is also serves a vital role in normal cycles of sleep and wakefulness—called circadian rhythms—that govern our 24-hour day. Histamine is produced in the brain in higher concentrations during the day, which keeps us awake and alert. Levels fall at night. If histamine production is stimulated at night, as is sometimes the case when mosquitoes or spiders bite us, it not only itches, but can keep you awake. We will discuss antihistamines later in the book but, briefly, they are distinguished by the fact that some make us sleepy and some don't. The ones that make us sleepy suppress both the histamine making us sneeze, and the histamine in the brain that keeps us awake. That is why some antihistamines can be used while driving and some cannot.

Beyond Histamine

Almost forty years ago, the chemistry of allergy began to change with the research of Dr. Frank Austin of Harvard. He observed that within the mast cell was not just histamine but also a "soup" of other "granular" substances that operate on different schedules from histamine.

Austin found that in addition to the ready-made histamine, the mast cells manufacture new mediators from the stored substances over a period of three to four hours. Many years later, these were identified as what we now call *leukotrienes*. They are dispersed into the surrounding area, where they contribute to inflammation, damaging otherwise healthy tissue long after the histamine has done its work.

We are just learning how to treat the problems associated with this next phase. The chemicals released by the mast cells are involved

---

DR. AUSTIN'S MAST CELL SOUP

The following is a list of the known mediators in a mast cell:
Preformed mediators—histamine, tryptase, chymase, chondroitin sulfate, carboxypeptidase A, cathepsin G, acid hydrolase, heparin.
Newly Synthesized Lipids—LTC4, A4, B4, D4, E4, PAF, PGD2.
Cytokines—IL-3, -4, -5, -6, -8, -10, -13, -16, TNF-α, MIP-1α, GM-CSF, β-FGF, SCF, TGF-β, VEGF, VPF, RANTES, MCP.

If you want to know what all these things mean, see page 32 of *Atlas of Allergic Diseases* by Phillip L. Lieberman and Michael S. Blaiss.

---

in the accumulation of inflammatory cells—*platelets, neutrophils*, and especially *eosinophils*—that are associated with the production of a variety of *cytokines* and adhesion molecules.

Cytokines—small proteins that influence immune response, although their role in allergic inflammation is difficult to pin down—are made not only in mast cells and basophils but also in practically any cell directly or indirectly involved in the allergic response. To complicate things still further, they can cause inflammation or can be anti-inflammatory.

Most recently, research documenting the role adhesion molecules play in allowing cells to stop and do their work in particular parts of the body has added another dimension to our understanding of allergic disease. The development of new medications that interfere with the action of cytokines and cellular adhesion molecules is the focus of current research.

Building on Dr. Austin's work, science is now delineating a tertiary stage of allergy toxicity that might be described as cellular destruction. It is not fully understood at this time, let alone treatable. But we can say with reasonable certainty that the more healthy tissue is subject to allergic inflammation, the more likely it is to sustain permanent damage. Therefore, we must do everything we can to avert allergic attack in the first place, and then to minimize its severity.

The allergic response is a cyclical process with escalating consequences. Our clinical focus now, and the focus of science in the future, will be to interrupt the process at the earliest possible moment, so as to minimize the long-term dangers.

However, our purpose here is not to explicate the frontiers of scientific discovery. It's to help you understand what you can do to help minimize the misery your child must endure, and to do that, we are going to try to stay away from the terminology of science and put our information in accessible language.

We realize that we have resorted to analogies repeatedly in this chapter, using guard dogs and police actions. We are going to use one more to describe these three stages. This time it's the military. We don't do this lightly at a time when U.S. troops are stationed in hostile lands. People resort to military analogies to describe everything from football to such brave business strategies as firing people by the thousands.

However, we believe that allergies can be a life-or-death matter and so justify the use of military comparisons. Furthermore, they are

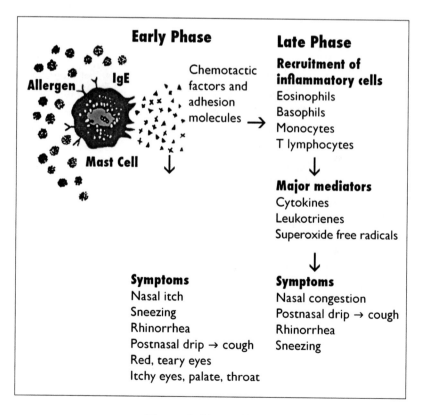

Figure 3. Mast cell soup

particularly apt and vivid, and we will use them later in the book as we refer to this chapter.

Think of that first phase of allergy as the reconnaissance phase, when special operations forces parachute into enemy territory, find command centers and blow them up, find out where to land the other troops, and target strategic facilities for attack.

The second phase is the infantry and aerial bombardment, when the enemy is destroyed but there's grave danger of collateral damage to innocent tissue.

The third phase is the unknown, when land mines and unexploded bombs are left behind, when snipers and saboteurs remain underground, and when the civilian population struggles to recover from the damage. We allergists win our wars, but we have to ask ourselves, Are we winning the peace? It's a much harder question to answer.

Why My Child?

Why are some people "tolerant" to allergens, e.g., why can they be exposed to the same antigens as the allergic individual without even noticing it? Why do others become truly "immune" to substances that are literally life threatening to the allergic?

We can't really say.

But if you think about allergy again as a survival from the days when people needed IgE to fight off parasites, you might get a clue. An allergic agent that once had to fight off a worm that grew on the banks of the Tigris and Euphrates rivers—the "Cradle of Civilization"—would have needed some powerful toxins to accomplish its task. Or an African tribe might have needed some other toxins to fight off parasites borne by flies. Some people were better at producing IgE. This might have made the difference between surviving and not surviving parasitic infection. So the descendants owe the existence of their hereditary line to this ability, which lay dormant in their genes through thousands of years of migration. Yet when these people are exposed to the fruits of modern living, like air-conditioning and modern bedding, or to unaccustomed vegetation, or household pets, those once-benign bodily mechanisms reemerge.

DOUBLE TROUBLE

Before we fully understood Dr. Austin's mast cell soup, we focused on only one ingredient, histamine, which causes severe immediate allergic reactions. We overlooked that this soup also contained what Dr. Austin called slow reactive substances of anaphylaxis (SRS-A). These mast cell products cause a late-phase reaction about twelve hours after exposure. The allergic victim may have both an immediate and late reaction.

Frank, who loved golf almost more than living, demonstrated to me that occasionally, a late-phase reaction could overshadow the immediate one. He got stung by a yellow jacket on Saturday and had a severe allergic reaction on Sunday. A trip to another allergist revealed no immediate skin-test reactions to yellow jackets. Frank returned to his golf. A second yellow-jacket sting resulted in a second late-phase reaction.

When I tested Frank for yellow jacket, I too found no immediate reaction. Some extra sense prompted me to ask Frank what happened to his yellow-jacket skin test after about twelve hours on the first session.

"As a matter of fact, they blew up and itched like hell. When I called the other allergist, he said to pay them no mind."

I said, "Frank, come back so I can see the tests tomorrow."

They were positive. Frank was worried. "How serious is this, Doc? I've heard that bee-sting allergy can be fatal. When I told my wife I would rather die than give up golf, I didn't mean it literally."

I began a series of yellow-jacket venom injections starting at a dose equivalent to one-millionth of a sting up to a maintenance dose equal to two stings.

Frank returned to his beloved golf and yellow-jacket stings. This time he had no reactions—not even late-phase ones. But it did nothing for his golf game.

— *Dr. Chiaramonte*

Safety, or Danger, in Numbers

The severity of the attack will depend on the concentration of mast cells and basophils at the point of exposure. The concentration in skin, for example, is low, and the flow of blood limited, which prevents large numbers of mast cells from other parts of the body from getting to the site. Therefore, a topical exposure—on the skin—will likely produce an uncomfortable but not dangerous response. This is also why allergy testing is done on the skin: Even with life-threatening sensitivities, the danger of skin testing is fairly minor because of the low concentrations of mast cells.

More dangerous are allergens that are inhaled or ingested, because they find their way to more critical parts of the body, such as the lungs. Furthermore, because blood flow to these areas is so much better than to the skin, more mast cells and other "reinforcements" arrive very quickly to help in the fight. The resulting inflammation when they spring into action can be life-threatening.

Inflammation—The Enemy at All Levels

The most dangerous allergic response is chronic inflammation, which can damage tissue cumulatively wherever it occurs. The antibodies attack the intruder and in the process draw other tissues—cells and fluids—to the afflicted area. This is what makes an infected cut swell and turn red, makes the nose run during pollen season, or makes an asthmatic wheeze. Acute symptoms subside in time, but there are both short- and long-term dangers.

The danger depends on the level of inflammation. All that attraction of fluids and other substances can kill during an asthma attack or anaphylactic shock, but short of that, they can also damage the affected tissues, rendering them less capable of performing their normal functions.

A child might scratch a bite until it bleeds and leave a scar, for example. That's why it's important to provide short-term relief of pain for minor allergens. But even without scratching, such skin conditions as hives might produce scarring, so it's important to control inflammation even for fundamentally minor allergens.

One problem is that the same medications that are most effective for controlling inflammation, steroids, have side effects of their own. Anyone who has used topical steroids—skin creams—for eczema or other conditions knows that, over a period of time, the skin will grow thinner, more like scar tissue than healthy skin. We are especially careful when the inflammation is on the face, because the skin is thinner, and damage is highly visible. Yet in the short run, relief from itching and flaking is worth it.

The practice of allergy medicine involves continual monitoring of the level of inflammation and weighing the dangers of inflammation against the consequences of treatment.

Latin Lesson

In medical school we learn that inflammation is characterized by four things:

Rubor—Color or redness generated by the increased blood flow into a region.

Tumor—Swelling caused by the release of fluid from the blood vessels in the region.

Dolor—Pain, as increased swelling stimulates local pain fibers.

Calor—Heat, as increased blood flow generates heat.

When you look at these words in the context of modern English, you can appreciate the many characteristics ascribed to these symptoms of inflammation:

Rubor—Think of ruby red, the color of blood.

Tumor—What does tumor mean in old English? It's a swelling on the body, either cancerous or not.

Dolor—Pain.

Calor—Calories are units of energy, and energy gives off what? Heat.

Clearly, inflammation was serious business to the Roman doctors, and it's serious now. Inflammation is not the cause of allergy, but it is the most serious recurring symptom. What happens to your child's skin if a cut goes untreated? The redness, the swelling, and the pain as cells from all over your body congregate to fight the infection—it can look pretty alarming. Now imagine the same thing happening in your child's sinuses. Just because you can't see the inflammation doesn't mean your child isn't suffering.

CHAPTER 3

What Is Asthma?

STHMA IS A MOVING TARGET. WHEEZING AND SHORTNESS OF breath—what doctors call "paroxysmal reversible airway obstruction"—have always been the symptoms that we equate with an asthma attack, but now we know that an attack is much more than this. These symptoms come and go and are usually reversible with medications.

But the problems don't stop there, of course. After the attack subsides, and apparently normal breathing is restored, the asthma is still there. Inflammation, caused by the movement of specialized white blood cells into the lining of the airways, produces swelling.

Asthma can be compared to a pot of water boiling on a stove. Inflammation is the burner underneath the pot. When the asthma gets severe, the pot boils over into an attack. For many years, treatment has focused on reopening the airways and ending the symptoms—in effect turning down the temperature and making sure the water doesn't spill over the sides of the pot.

However, alleviating these symptoms doesn't mean that the heat has been turned off. The residual inflammation may just be simmering under the pot. Just as the lower heat will eventually cause the liquid in the pot to evaporate and damage the pot itself, chronic inflammation can lead to permanent changes in the airways called *remodeling*. Remodeling can make what was once reversible obstruction into permanent damage.

The Paradox of Allergic Inflammation

From the above description, it may sound as though inflammation is a bad thing, but it's really a good thing. The inflammatory process is vital for helping fight infection. With allergy and asthma, however, in which inflammation is fighting an otherwise harmless enemy, it is bad.

Unfortunately, the regular use of anti-inflammatory medication for fighting "bad" inflammation will also interfere with "good" inflammation, the inflammatory process that seeks to deal with real bacterial or viral infection. The use of a helpful drug like prednisone, for example, which is generally taken orally, will eventually hurt the functioning of the larger immune system. The relief you experience from itching or other symptoms may be worth it, at least for a time. This trade-off is a fact of life for asthmatics and their doctors, and it is one reason that we welcome the further development of anti-inflammatory medicines that can be delivered locally to the lungs, since their effects on other parts of the body that might be infected are limited.

Hyperresponsive Airways

Most asthmatics have very sensitive, hyperresponsive airways. Their airways narrow after exposure to very small amounts of irritants like smoke, or allergens like pollen or dust.

Some have airways that react to exposure to cold air or to exercise, which will be discussed in more detail in chapter 4. Stress is also a factor. As you can see, like all of allergy, asthma is a complex condition. There is no single test to diagnose it. A doctor must take into account the patient's entire history, physical examination, and both laboratory and breathing tests.

The Closest Thing to a Sure Test

The closest procedure to a sure test for asthma is to *challenge* the patient with a substance called *methacholine*, a chemical that triggers *bronchospasm* in almost anyone when inhaled in large doses. The asthmatic patient is sensitive to even tiny doses. This can help a doctor to identify people at risk of developing asthma.

This test is time consuming because measures must be taken to avoid a full-grown asthma attack. A new alternative is measuring exhaled nitric oxide (eNO), which indicates airway inflammation, a test that can be done in minutes without the risk of an attack. It has only recently become available on a practical level.

This is not the same as *nitrous* oxide, or laughing gas. Nitric oxide is higher in people whose lungs are inflamed, as they are with asthma. You can be asymptomatic and still have inflammation at destructive levels. We have long been able to measure exhaled nitric oxide, but until fairly recently the equipment to do so was prohibitively expensive. A Swedish company called Aerocrine (which, in the interest of full disclosure, Dr. Ehrlich has worked with) now makes a low-cost portable device called NIOX MINO that more medical offices can afford to buy.

Both authors and others now use this device to assess asthma severity and control. The eNO measurement can also be used to reduce dosages of inhaled steroids more precisely when inflammation levels warrant.

A competing product made by Apieron is the Insight eNO System.

Naughty or Nice?

Taking your medication to control chronic disease, along with the behavioral instructions the doctor gives you, is called compliance, or adherence. Thus, for example, an asthmatic with an allergy to cats will be told to take his meds and stay away from cats. We will talk more about compliance in chapter 8.

Hard as it is to believe, many asthmatics, as well as other patients who have chronic disease, do not take their medicine as directed, which is one of the reasons that patients of all ages end up in emergency rooms, or worse. Moreover, these patients will lie about it, to their parents, and to their doctors. With the march of technology, however, we can now tell.

Doctors can use the eNO device to confront patients who swear up and down that they are taking their medicine. If the eNO levels are high, we know it's a lie. Faced with the evidence, they will 'fess up. It has saved lives.

A teenage boy with severe persistent asthma had been hospitalized twenty-seven times, including three times in the ICU, with intubation, and missed many days of school. He lived with his mother and a wheelchair-bound sister. He had been treated by his referring pediatrician with oral steroids, high-dose inhaled steroids, and a drugstore full of other medications, yet he did not get better. Long-term high-dose steroid use had resulted in bone demineralization.

A specialist suspected noncompliance, but the records showed otherwise. The mother had filled the prescriptions regularly and the many residents and nurses who had seen the boy in the hospital were convinced he was compliant.

The doctor was on the verge of notifying the state health department that the boy was at risk of imminent death. But NIOX MINO technology showed an eNO level of 78. Faced with the evidence of elevated inflammation, the patient confessed to systematically hiding the medication under his bed, where it was found. Resuming his high-dose oral steroids, his eNO levels came down to 17. He was then weaned to low-dose inhaled steroids, and his eNO levels stabilized at 11. He has had no more medical emergencies or school absences.

Why would a boy jeopardize his own life in this way? Good question. It surely had to do with his family situation. Family dynamics are complicated when one child has a condition that takes a disproportionate amount of parental attention, although it's usually the asthmatic child who gets it. Suffice it to say for now, this needy boy received the necessary psychological support along with his medical treatment. We discuss this subject further in chapter 14.

Unfortunately, many nonspecialists concentrate just on the outward symptoms of asthma, and prescribe medication that relieves them. Even when the symptoms are in abeyance, however, underlying inflammation may be causing permanent damage.

SOCCER AND THE REAL TEST FOR ASTHMA

I had a 10-year-old patient, who was referred to me by a pediatrician, and who complained that he had to see a specialist.

"I'm fine," he said. "Don't have any trouble. I take my medicine and when I start to wheeze, I take a quick hit from my inhaler." I listened to his chest and his lungs were certainly clear.

"I had to miss soccer practice to come in here," he said, looking at his mother.

"Great game," I said. "That's a good sign. Takes a lot of energy. What position do you play?"

"Halfback," he answered. "Well, I'm really a halfback but they switched me to goalie." — *Dr. Ehrlich*

Sometimes a simple piece of information is a better indicator of an asthmatic condition than anything we can do clinically. For there it was in a neat package. From halfback, where you have to run your tail off, to goalie, where you don't. You can see the child's identity changing. "I'm really a halfback." Certainly there are worse outcomes in asthma treatment, but there are also better ones, and we grown-ups—doctors and parents—don't always find them or strive for them. The patients—children—suffer.

Treating asthma is often a question of these in-between values, a kind of no-man's-land of conflicting physiological and psychological issues. Many general practitioners and pediatricians are experts at treating the overt, alarming aspects of the disease, but they fall short on the supposedly lesser ones, which is where the most damage

---

CHECKLIST TO HELP DIAGNOSE ASTHMA IN SCHOOL-AGED CHILDREN

Does the child...

Make noisy or wheezy sounds when breathing?
Have a hard time taking a deep breath?
Develop coughs that won't go away?
Complain about chest tightness or pain after running?
Have trouble breathing when running?
Cough when running?
Have a hard time breathing in cold weather?
Wake up at night coughing?
Wake up at night because of trouble breathing?
Have itchy, puffy, or burning eyes?
Have problems with a runny, stuffy nose?
Miss days of school because of breathing problems?
Cough around pets?
Have trouble breathing around pets?
Have difficulty with foods?

Has the child...

Been told he or she has asthma or bronchitis?
Been hospitalized or taken medicines for asthma or bronchitis?
— Adapted from the American College of Allergy, Asthma & Immunology questionnaire

---

is probably done. They are even reluctant to use the A-word, *asthma*, because it is alarming to parents. But denial is counterproductive. A wait-and-see attitude is a recipe for chronic inflammation and permanent damage to the airways. It does no good to call wheezing—or chronic coughing for that matter—bronchitis. Make sure your little halfback can remain a halfback

Sleep/Work/Play—
Three Questions About Your Child's Quality of Life

During the past few years, we worked with the Asthma and Allergy Foundation of America (AAFA) to help establish a new diagnostic tool that centers on the quality of a child's life. It boils down to three simple questions:

- Do you sleep tight?
- Do you work right?
- Do you play with might?

This sleep-work-play model was for a time the basis of an AAFA-affiliated website, but the fact that it has disappeared from the web is by no means an indicator that its usefulness has slipped away, and that is why we are going to recap it here.

Each of these questions reflects a key signal of illness and health as it pertains to asthma.

Quality of sleep is not just about the more than eight hours a night a healthy child spends in dreamland. A child who coughs and wheezes and wakes through the night will be sluggish and inattentive at school. In fact, the science of sleep medicine shows that the symptoms teachers and parents use to determine whether a child has attention deficit hyperactivity disorder (ADHD) are almost identical to those of sleep deprivation. It is estimated that half of children who are being treated for ADHD really should have their sleep evaluated. To the extent that your asthmatic child is having trouble in school, it is worth making sure that the truly treatable condition is treated conscientiously. It is disturbing to think that millions of parents who are shy of steroids and lax about other allergy control measures may be medicating their children with Aderall or Ritalin because they aren't paying attention in school.

SLEEP, ASTHMA, ALLERGIES

These are facts I cite in my lectures to doctors (as printed in *Sleep to Save Your Life* by Dr. Gerard Lombardo):

• Disruption of nighttime sleep impairs daytime wakefulness, cognitive functioning, psychomotor speed and coordination, and mood.
• Children with perennial allergic rhinitis have significant sleep disturbance.
• In a study of fifty-four first graders with obstructive sleep apnea, twenty-four underwent tonsillectomy and adenoidectomy.
The mean grades of treated students during the second grade increased significantly. No academic improvement occurred in the untreated group.
• The presence of nasal congestion associated with allergic rhinitis is a risk factor for obstructive sleep apnea.
• A study of thirty-nine children with habitual snoring found the frequency of obstructive sleep apnea was 50 percent greater for allergic than nonallergic subjects.
• A survey of 400 parents with allergic and nonallergic children found that allergic children were significantly more withdrawn and drowsy.
• A common problem in allergic rhinitis is inflammation and fluid in the Eustachian tubes, the tubes that go from the nasopharynx to the middle ear, which was found to be strongly related to inattentiveness and over-talkativeness.

Dr. Ehrlich

We must point out that any blockage in the upper airways, whether from mucus, inflammation, or being overweight, can affect nighttime breathing, resulting in snoring or sleep apnea, which is the cessation of breathing. These are very bad for anyone. The body compensates by activation of the "flight or fight response," the extra gear nature gave us to fight our enemies or run away from predators. It is very taxing on the body. Blood pressure rises precipitously. The adrenal glands go into overdrive—it's like having to use your rescue inhaler hundreds of times in a night. No wonder you're so miserable in the morning: You have nothing left!

This is a terrible, life-threatening condition for adults. For children it is an unfair handicap with lifelong implications.

What Happens During an Asthma Attack?
The Doctor's Version

The lungs are composed of various specialized cells and tissues—not just simple tubes or pipes. Lining them are epithelial cells with specialized hairs, or cilia, which help trap particles and prevent infection from reaching the lungs. They also help push foreign and waste matter out of the lungs when necessary. Beneath these cells is the

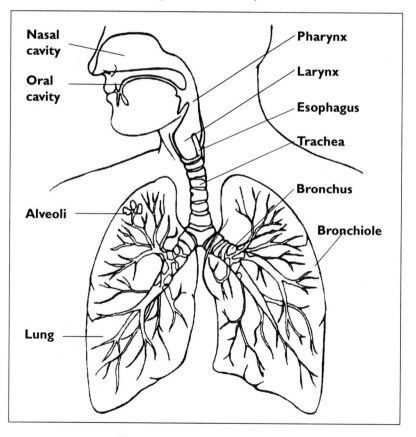

Figure 4. The respiratory system

"basement membrane" that forms a firm foundation for the epithelial cells, and under that is looser tissue full of mucous glands and other specialized cells such as eosinophils, mast cells, lymphocytes, and white blood cells called polys. Under this layer is smooth muscle. During an asthma attack the epithelial cells are sloughed off, which in turn helps thicken the mucus and plugs up the airways. The other cells release chemicals, or mediators, which attract additional white blood cells that damage the tissues or cause the smooth muscle to constrict. These actions combine to narrow the airways and obstruct breathing. It is useful to understand that the problem with asthma is not only that it is difficult to *inhale,* it is difficult to fully *exhale.* Air that is ready to be exhaled is full of carbon dioxide, and when it remains in the lungs, it can produce light-headedness, panic, and eventual unconsciousness.

What Happens During an Asthma Attack?
The Parent's Version

While the first signs of impending asthma may differ in each child, the common signs are feelings of pressure in the chest, itchiness in places that can't be scratched (such as inside the rib cage), breathlessness, elongation of the time it takes to exhale, and the overall process of breathing becoming more rapid and labored. The particular symptoms for individual children seem to repeat themselves. One 60-year-old we know can still recall his first-ever asthma attack when he was 12. "I suddenly felt, and sounded, like an accordion. I had no idea what was happening to me."

Wheezing, that whistling sound most closely associated with asthma, is actually a symptom of an attack that has advanced beyond the earliest stages. It is usually preceded by a dry cough, and the wheezing itself is generally heard only at the end of exhalation. The child can talk in sentences, although with some difficulty, and may want to lie down to breathe more comfortably. At this point the breathing may be slightly labored as the respiratory muscles are not retracting. Some signs of agitation may accompany the rapid breathing and prolonged exhalation at this mild stage.

"GOOD" STEROIDS AND "BAD" STEROIDS

Parents are fearful of steroids because athletes give them a bad name. LET'S GET THIS PERFECTLY CLEAR: The only thing your child's asthma medicine has in common with "performance enhancing" drugs is the name. Your child's medicine is an anti-inflammatory *corticosteroid*, derived from the adrenal cortex, the outer layer of the adrenal glands. It won't enlarge any body parts or grow hair where it shouldn't be.

They are NOT the same as *anabolic steroids*, which turn 97-pound weaklings into the Incredible Hulk or Jose Canseco, and are derived from testosterone.

The peak flow rate—air flow out measured by a simple device, which we will explain in greater detail later on—will be about 80 percent of the child's best measurement.

Moderate Asthma Attack

The attack we just described was mild, and should be treatable at home by an experienced family. However, when an attack progresses beyond the mild stage, the child will prefer to sit up to breathe, become more agitated, and talk in phrases, rather than full sentences. Breathing will be more rapid, as exhaling takes longer and becomes more labored. The wheezing sound will be loud, extending throughout exhalation with visible action of the muscles of the chest and neck.

At this point, the peak flow has fallen to between 50 and 80 percent of the child's best measurement and treatment should be given by doctors, probably in the ER, or at least in the presence of a physician. Steroids are injected to reduce inflammation because inhaled steroids, whether in powdered form or in nebulized aerosol form, might not make it into the lungs because of mucus and other airway blockages. The steroids will take at least four hours to work. Bronchodilators—drugs inhaled to relax the

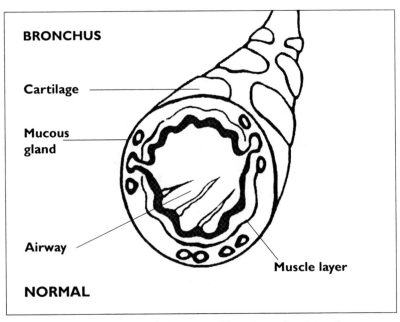

BRONCHUS

Cartilage

Mucous gland

Airway

Muscle layer

NORMAL

Everything is in its place and behaving itself, so the air has lots of room to come and go.

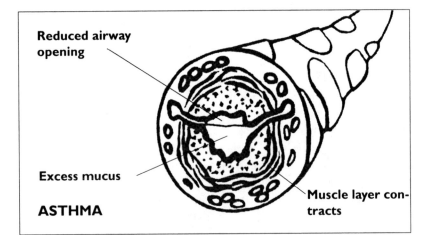

Reduced airway opening

Excess mucus

ASTHMA

Muscle layer contracts

The airways start going into lockdown. The muscles contract and mucus fills the airway, making it much more difficult for fresh oxygen-rich air to get to the lungs and the spent carbon dioxide–rich air to get out.

Figure 5. Asthma illustrated

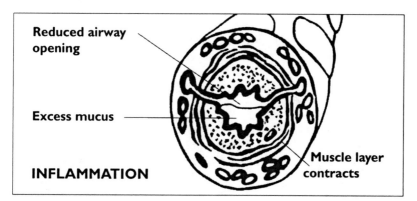

Reduced airway opening

Excess mucus

INFLAMMATION

Muscle layer contracts

The inflammatory stage. All those allergy-fighting mechanisms are in full swing. Eosinophils, basophils, and other cells are accumulating along with the fluid that carries them, and they are releasing leukotrienes, cytokines, and other mediators. Remember our little Latin lesson? *Rubor*—ruby red color; *Tumor*—swelling; *Dolor*—pain; *Calor*—heat. All these are taking place in those delicate tissues. Upon repeated incidence, the tissues will undergo a permanent change callled *airway remodeling*. Imagine an acne scar on your child's airways! Don't let it happen! Make sure he or she uses the anti-inflammatory medication!

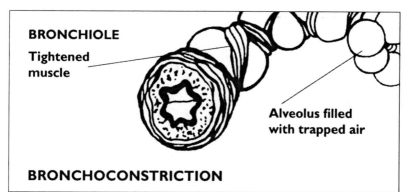

BRONCHIOLE

Tightened muscle

Alveolus filled with trapped air

BRONCHOCONSTRICTION

Life-threatening. Fresh air can't get in, and spent air can't get out. And look at what is happening to those delicate bronchioles! What happens to a balloon after you blow it up and tie it off? Think of your child's birthday parties. Those balloons don't look so good the next day. You can't just untie them and blow them up again, good as new. Think of that drab rubber as the delicate, microscopically thin tissue, where oxygen is exchanged for carbon dioxide.

smooth muscles in the airway that become constricted during an attack—will be given. An intravenous infusion of steroids and fluids may be started, along with oxygen.

Severe Asthma Attack

By this point, the child sits upright and is very agitated, speaking in words only. The shoulders are hunched over, and every chest, neck, and stomach muscle is enlisted in the struggle to breathe. Very loud wheezing now extends throughout the breathing cycle, both inhalation and exhalation, with a rapid respiratory rate. Bronchodilators, steroids, intravenous fluids, and oxygen should have been given to the child in the emergency room or hospital by now. The peak flow will be less than 50 percent of the child's best. Blood gases—oxygen and carbon dioxide—will be abnormal even if oxygen is being administered.

Impending Respiratory Arrest

The work of breathing has become too much for the by-now drowsy and confused child.

WARNING: If there is no wheezing, then not enough air is being moved through the bronchi to make any noise.

RED ALERT: In fact, there are no breath sounds. The carbon dioxide rises, increasing the acid in the blood. The blood oxygen falls rapidly and only at this late stage does the child turn blue. Keeping the child alive requires being in the intensive care unit with assisted respiration.

Who Gets Asthma?

Dr. Anthony Gagliardi, a pulmonologist at St. Vincent's Hospital in New York, says that the study of asthma "is the study of one." That is, asthma describes a set of symptoms—also known as "asthma syndrome," which we discuss later in this chapter—that may be triggered by many allergic or environmental causes, or, by Dr. Martin's reckoning, bacterial infection. We have to solve the mysteries, and treat them, one at a time.

SOUNDS OF SILENCE

More years ago than I would like to admit, I was a supervising resident of a large city hospital that served poor children primarily. I worked with interns, doctors just out of medical school. It was a balancing act: protecting the children from less experienced doctors while giving these interns room to gain experience and learn. We all worked long hours through many sleepless nights.

Sometimes snap judgments had to be made during those long shifts. But I always told my interns, "When in doubt, ask." Dr. Kramer was a shy but better-than-average intern. She called me one morning in tears. "They admitted a 12-year-old asthmatic boy to my service at ten last night. I started treatment and went on to another admission. When I returned to check on him a few minutes ago he was dead."

That morning I reviewed the chart, and talked to the mother.

Many high-risk factors had been missed upon admission during a very busy night. Among them, the boy had a recent hospitalization for asthma, and had been seen in several different emergency rooms over the preceding few days, also for asthma. In addition, use of oral steroids had recently been stopped, and someone forgot to tell Dr. Kramer that the boy had been intubated (had a breathing tube inserted by mouth) for asthma in the past. He was also using his bronchodilator repeatedly without his inhaled steroids, which is a lopsided, medically risky way to treat chronic asthma that is no longer allowed.

Not learning all this was a tragic oversight, although if you ever see a New York City emergency room on a Saturday night, you will find it credible. But Dr. Kramer's real mistake was one of well-intentioned judgment. The child was lying in a dark open ward, and the doctor didn't turn on a light so as not to awaken the other children. She didn't hear any wheezing and took that as a sign that the treatment was working. She learned the hard way that sometimes the absence of wheezing is a bad sign, not a good one.   — *Dr. Chiaramonte*

Although no single "asthma gene" has been discovered, asthma does seem to run in families. Asthma also tends to occur more often in families that have a history of other allergies, and in fact, many patients have both asthma and allergies of the nose, eyes, or skin.

If a parent or sibling has asthma, there is greater likelihood of *early-onset asthma*, which means it develops early in childhood. If the parents smoke, particularly the mother, it increases the incidence of asthma at a young age. Still, asthma may start at any age. Attacks are triggered by substances to which children are allergic. For example, a patient with cat allergy develops an asthma attack when he visits a home with cats.

Obesity, exposure to fumes, irritants such as tobacco smoke, or rapid changes in temperature and humidity levels from going in and out of air-conditioned buildings during a hot summer can be asthma triggers. Other risk factors include gastroesophageal reflux disease (GERD), which many people have learned about from recent television advertising, although it is fairly common and no joke to those who suffer from it. Reflux occurs when stomach contents come back up the esophagus, or swallowing tube. These juices can either spill into the lung or irritate nerves in the esophagus. Chronic infections can also contribute to development of asthma. Bacterial lung infections have been linked to asthma.

At the Asthma Research Center in Denver, Dr. Richard Martin and his colleagues are expanding and clarifying the concept that infection plays a key role in the origin of chronic asthma, at least in some people. During the past four years, they have firmly established that *Mycoplasma* and *Chlamydia*, two kinds of bacteria that are very common and often cause pneumonia, are present in the airways of a large subset of asthmatics. This is intriguing research by a first-class doctor at a first-class institution, but it is a work in progress, so the clinical payoff, if any, remains years away.

Chronic sinus infection is associated with asthma attacks in some people. Their sinuses are inflamed. Some asthma patients develop sensitivity to aspirin and other nonsteroidal anti-inflammatory drugs such as ibuprofen and naproxen, and they tend to develop nasal polyps—mucous growths in the mucous membranes. Their asthma may be very difficult to manage.

Asthma and Bronchitis—The Name Game

Bronchitis, a term that refers to inflammation in the bronchi or larger airways of the lungs, may be due to infection or other immune processes in the lungs, not asthma. While the symptoms of bronchitis may overlap with those of asthma, bronchitis does not typically cause the airway obstruction that is the characteristic of asthma. An asthmatic cough is usually *productive*, that is, sputum is brought up, whereas a bronchial cough is *nonproductive*, with no sputum.

The confusion between bronchitis and asthma is fertile ground for misunderstanding and imprecise language. For example, "bronchial asthma" is actually a redundant term since the bronchi are always involved in asthma.

Some doctors refer to "asthmatic bronchitis" or "reactive airway disease" when a patient is having trouble breathing and perhaps wheezing, but they are not sure if the patient is suffering from an ongoing condition. This is often the case with infants and small children who start to wheeze when suffering from viral infections such as respiratory syncytial virus. Many may wheeze just once when they've had a viral respiratory infection, or occasionally over a period of one or two years. Some, however, do go on to develop classic asthma.

Patients or their parents may be concerned about having the diagnosis of "asthma" entered into their medical records because they fear that insurance companies may require higher premiums or refuse to insure them. Some young people fear that the diagnosis may prevent them from playing varsity sports or serving in the military. Unfortunately, the use of other names for asthma does not avoid these problems. It also complicates the problem of administering effective treatment, both short- and long-term. And finally, an inaccurate medical record can lead to mistaken, fatal treatment in emergency circumstances.

Coughing and Wheezing

Painful as it can be, a cough is the body's way of protecting the lungs by clearing the airways of foreign material. Most asthmatics cough at some point in an attack. If the cough triggers airway spasm or tightness, or is continuous, it can be harmful.

Some attacks start with a cough that becomes progressively tighter, and is then followed by wheezing. However, some asthmatics just begin wheezing without coughing. While it usually requires a stethoscope or a trained ear to the chest to hear the wheezing, when it becomes more severe the patient and those around him will hear it too.

Still, some asthmatics never wheeze during attacks but only cough. They suffer from so-called *cough-variant asthma*, which occurs when inflammation and bronchoconstriction are concentrated in parts of the airways, not spread generally throughout them as they would be in what might be deemed "normal" asthma. Think of them as "sleeper cells" that can provoke general trouble for the whole body, as the patient is wracked with extended coughing episodes. The coughing is the body's effort to expel these local troublemakers, as if they were actual physical entities, such as dust or particles of dirt. We must treat to control the underlying inflammation as we would with the more familiar wheezing.

Mucus Rising

Normally thin and watery, mucus traps bacteria or pollen or dust or other foreign particles. The cilia lining the airways then help push the mucus up and out of the lungs. This is the so-called "mucociliary escalator." During asthma attacks this escalator is like the escalators at the New York City subway station at 52nd Street and Lexington Avenue: It doesn't work very well. The mucus turns dry and hard, partly due to the labored breathing common in asthma attacks. It thickens as cells such as eosinophils, ciliated epithelial cells, polys, and lymphocytes die off and clog the airway. This thick, dry mucus in turn makes it harder for cilia to push up the foreign substances, and at the same time, the cilia themselves are rendered less effective as the ciliated cells themselves die and slough off.

As the airways begin to relax and breathing becomes easier, some patients begin to cough up mucus. Patients should thin this mucus as much as possible by drinking lots of fluids during an attack.

Contrary to conventional wisdom, steam and vaporizers are not usually very helpful in asthma attacks, since the large water droplets they form will not reach the lower airways where mucus creates the biggest problems. Some medicines, like guaifenesin and steroids, can also help thin mucus. In addition, bronchodilators can relax the smooth muscle of the airways and help open them up. When this happens, it becomes easier to exhale and cough up the mucus. In severe bouts, however, the mucus can completely block the airways—sometimes fatally.

CONCRETE PROBLEM

No one who has ever witnessed the autopsy of an asthma patient can ever forget the sight of the mucous plug that emerges from the lungs, the thing that has made breathing literally impossible.

When I was a resident, I watched as a pathologist withdrew a mucous plug almost as hard as concrete from the chest of a young boy. The lining of the airways was stuck to the mucus.

— *Dr. Chiaramonte*

LIQUID ASSETS

In my work with Project E.R.A.S.E., a nonprofit venture I founded with my friend Barbara Cutler to send asthma specialists directly to New York City public schools, I encourage parents to call me directly if their children are exhibiting emergency symptoms. One Saturday I received a call from a mother whose child had gone to emergency rooms about once a month for years. I told her, "Get a 2-liter bottle of juice or soda, and make him drink it overnight, and call me in the morning." Sure enough, he was fine the next day. Good hydration is necessary to keep that mucus in a liquid state so the escalator can do its work.

By the way, for anyone who cares about the other kind of liquid assets, the nation's health care bill, should keep this story in mind. Cost of an ER visit? Maybe six hundred bucks. Hospitalization? Close to $7,000. Costs of a bottle of juice, or tap water for that matter? Well, you do that arithmetic. And for the price of two liters of soda, Dr. Chiaramonte's autopsy boy might have been a 40-year-old man today.

— *Dr. Ehrlich*

Mucous Plugs

We frequently resort to alarming, colorful language in this book, but since asthma is a matter of life and death, we feel that the more colorful the language, the more memorable it will be, and the lessons will be learned more indelibly. How then to describe a fatal mucous plug?

Go to a fish store and take a look at a whole raw squid. With apologies to all you Italian food mavens out there, a mucous plug is remarkably similar to your beloved calamari before it has been cut up, coated with batter and deep-fried.

Airway Spasm

The lungs resemble an upside-down tree. The "trunk" is called the *trachea*, which leads from the throat into the chest. The trachea narrows into "branches" called *bronchi*. They in turn taper down into "twigs" called *small bronchi* and then *bronchioles*. Last, there are "leaves"—small sacs called *alveoli* where the blood exchanges carbon dioxide for fresh oxygen.

All the bronchi are surrounded by smooth muscle along with mucous glands. When the smooth muscle contracts, it leads to constriction, or narrowing, of the airways. This *bronchoconstriction* contributes to the airway obstruction known as asthma. When constriction is severe, the patient starts to feel that she cannot breathe. The lungs, in turn, may not be able to supply the blood with as much fresh oxygen as the body needs.

The other factors are the *edema*, or swelling, of the lining of the airways, which can damage it, as well as the increase in mucus. The medicines called bronchodilators help to relax the muscle spasm and allow passage of more air through the airways. They are usually inhaled, but can also be given as a pill or liquid. In severe episodes, an injection of *epinephrine* may be given if inhalation is not sufficient. These medicines are called *rescue medicines* since they act to open up the airways almost immediately. Epinephrine is also used in the event of *anaphylaxis*.

Swelling and Damage to Airway Lining

Recent studies have shown that the smooth muscle surrounding the airways in asthmatics contains dramatically more mast cells than that of people without asthma. As with any allergic response (see chapter 2, "When Cells Attack") the chemicals in the mast cells, the *mediators*, not only prompt spasm of the muscle itself, but increase mucus production, and draw other cells to the area, leading to an inflammatory response. These cells and the mediators lead to the increase in "twitchiness" of the airways characteristic of the asthmatic's lung.

Airway Remodeling

Asthma can start at any age. The trigger can be allergens such as dust, dust mites, animal dander, foods or food additives, or molds. Once the airways have become overly reactive, however, an attack can be brought on by cold air, exercise, smoke exposure or strong odors, or even by emotional upsets.

Approximately half of children with asthma will eventually "outgrow" it at least temporarily. However, the symptoms can recur when they are adults, particularly if the allergies are untreated. For reasons we don't yet understand, early-onset asthma is more common in males, while late-onset (adolescence or later) is more common in females.

Apart from saving lives, our major concern is with permanent changes in the airways, which can continue even if the number of attacks diminishes or appears to stop altogether. Currently, we cannot easily determine if the airways are continuing to alter even after symptoms cease. Studies have shown loss of elasticity of the lungs in patients with moderate or severe asthma.

The loss of elasticity stems at least in part to what we might call the Arnold Schwarzenegger effect. The smooth muscles that line the airways—known, cleverly, as airway smooth muscles or ASM— normally get just the right amount of exercise to stay toned. However, when inflammation causes bronchoconstriction, those muscles are getting what amounts to a heavy workout, and like any other heavy exercise, the workout makes them muscle bound.

Reversible or Irreversible?

In the past, asthma was thought to be an entirely reversible process. Now it is recognized that with persistent asthma or hyperresponsive airways, the smooth muscles surrounding the air tubes not only grow thicker, the airway linings lose cilia, making them less able to filter incoming air, which spurs an increase in mast cells to fight allergens that previously were filtered out. Finally, the basement membrane underneath the mucosal layer becomes thicker and swells with many different kinds of cells.

If this process persists untreated, the once-reversible airway obstruction becomes fixed and irreversible. That's why we, along with many other allergists, feel that inhaled steroids—corticosteroids inhaled either as a powder or propelled under pressure—should be started earlier than we once did. These medications control swelling, reduce mucus production, and make the airways less "twitchy," or sensitive to asthma triggers.

The irreversible damage can be subtle. Patients may not suffer any obvious attacks—the pot never or rarely boils over—but tests can show that the amount of air moving in and out of the lungs gets lower with each passing year, depriving them of the oxygen their bodies need for maintenance and growth.

WHERE THERE'S HEAT, THERE MAY BE LIGHT

A new method called *bronchial thermoplasty* may someday give us the ability to reverse some of the damage from airway remodeling. A bronchoscopically placed probe applies radio frequency to the walls of the central airway. The heat generated in this way reduces the muscle mass produced by years of extra exertion. As you can imagine, heat treatment causes some collateral effects, although so far these appear temporary, and the benefits seem to outweigh the damage. However, it will be years before this will be anything like a mainstream treatment. Regardless, preventing airway remodeling in the first place by carefully managing asthma is the best course.

Children's lung function should increase steadily as they grow, but in asthmatics, lung growth may not keep pace with the rest of their bodies. Thus, such lung function tests are key to monitoring and treating childhood asthma. Current testing is not adequate to the task of predicting airway remodeling, but work is under way to develop new methods.

Early diagnosis and treatment are essential to prevent asthma from causing permanent damage to the lungs and to ensure that every child can enjoy his or her childhood, complete with sports, travel, and visiting friends.

OUTPATIENT MANAGEMENT
FOR PRIMARY CARE PHYSICIANS

ON VISIT ONE

Take detailed history
Do physical exam

If Asthma Now

Obstruction or no obstruction?
Review Medications
   Bronchodilator
   Anti-inflammatory agents
Patient and Family Education
   Teach use of peak flow meter
   1) Establish green, yellow, and red zones for individual patient
   2) Establish green, yellow, and red medical program
   (Note: These colors refer to levels of air flow. Green is "normal,"
   yellow indicates a moderate asthma attack, and red indicates
   a severe attack, as described earlier in the chapter. See also
   "Green, Yellow, and Red Days" in chapter 8.)

Evaluate the Need for Systemic Corticosteroids
   Prescription of prednisone, 20–40 milligrams, 5–10 days

If Asthma Recently

Baseline pulmonary function test
Bronchodilators
Anti-inflammatory agents
Patient and family education

If Asthma, No Symptoms

Explain about bronchodilators and anti-inflammatories
Environmental control
Patient and family education
Teach peak flow meter

ON VISIT TWO

Review peak flow readings
Review medications
Refer patient to allergy clinic for appropriate workup

Guidelines for Treatment

As we stated earlier, NIH guidelines are followed only half the time in treating asthma, which we believe contributes to the high percentage of cases that result in hospitalization and long-term lung damage. Therefore, we believe it's important that patients have some idea of what constitutes effective procedure. Primary care physicians we are acquainted with at one multispecialty practice in New York City use the following:

National Institutes of Health
Asthma and Allergy Treatment Guidelines

The National Heart, Lung, and Blood Institute, one of the National Institutes of Health, recommends that treatment for asthma include four components:

- Use of objective measures of lung function to assess the severity of asthma and to monitor the course of therapy
- Comprehensive pharmacological therapy to reverse and prevent airway inflammation, which is characteristic of asthma, as well as to treat airway narrowing
- Environmental control measures to avoid or eliminate factors that induce or trigger asthma exacerbations, including consideration of immunotherapy, which builds up the body's own allergy-fighting capacity, and is discussed in chapter 9
- Patient education that fosters a partnership among the patient, his or her family, and the clinician

When to Refer to an Allergist

Based on these recommendations and treatment-outcome studies, referral guidelines have been developed by a joint committee of the two leading, relevant academic institutions.

Asthma and Allergy Referral Guidelines of the
American College of Allergy, Asthma & Immunology, and the
American Academy of Allergy, Asthma & Immunology

The guidelines state that referral to an allergist for asthma treatment is indicated under the following conditions:

- When the patient's asthma is unstable. Uncontrolled asthma may be associated with widely variable pulmonary functions and possibly high morbidity and mortality. Early comprehensive intervention may prevent these unfortunate events. Such intervention should include development of a long-term treatment plan.

• When the patient's response to treatment is limited, incomplete, or very slow, and poor control interferes with the patient's quality of life

• When, in spite of taking anti-inflammatory medications regularly, the patient must use an inhaled beta-agonist such as albuterol frequently, exclusive of its use in exercise-induced asthma. Albuterol simulates beta-2 neurotransmitters and relaxes the bronchial muscles. (For more information on beta-agonists, see chapter 5.)

• If there is a need for frequent adjustments of therapy because of unstable asthma

• For identification of allergens or other environmental factors that may be causing the patient's disease. Patients with asthma must have access to a thorough etiologic evaluation. (*Etiologic* is a fancy name for the process of determining the cause of a disorder. For example, an etiologic evaluation of an allergy might reveal that there is a cat at home.)

• When allergen immunotherapy is a consideration

• When the patient and the primary caregiver need intensive education in the role of allergens and other environmental factors

• When family d0ynamics interfere with patient care and/or there is a need for further family education about asthma

• When a patient has a chronic cough that is refractory, or irresponsive, to usual therapy

• When coexisting illnesses and/or their treatment complicate the management of asthma

• When the patient has recurrent absences from school or work due to asthma

• When the patient is experiencing continuing, nocturnal episodes of asthma

• When the patient is unable to participate in normal daily activities or sports because of limited exercise ability despite use of inhaled beta-agonists prior to exercise

• When the patient requires multiple medications on a long-term basis

• When frequent bursts of oral corticosteroids or daily oral corticosteroids are required

• When the patient exhibits excessive liability of pulmonary function (shortage of breath), e.g., highly variable peak flow rates

- When the diagnosis of asthma is in doubt
- When there is concern about side effects that have occurred or may occur, e.g., use of oral or orally inhaled corticosteroids in children
- When preventive measures need to be considered for the high-risk, predisposed infant with a family history of asthma or atopy (allergy)
  - Sudden severe attacks of asthma
  - Hospitalization of the patient for asthma
  - Severe episodes of asthma resulting in loss of consciousness
  - Seizures, near-death episodes or respiratory failure requiring artificial respiration
  - When emergency room visits are required to control the patient's asthma
  - When the patient asks for a consultation

Asthma Syndrome, Nonallergic Asthma, and COPD

While these aren't strictly within the scope of this book, we would like to say a bit about them because they are entering common parlance and are very likely to confuse diagnosis and treatment of asthma in years to come. We have come to see that allergic asthma is just one of the contributors to a set of symptoms. These symptoms are now called asthma syndrome, and they have all been described here. One way to distinguish between a disease and a syndrome is to consider the case of Muhammad Ali, who suffers from Parkinson's *Syndrome*, not Parkinson's *Disease*. That is, he exhibits the symptoms associated with the disease, but the damage to his brain came from getting punched in the head many times, not from a genetic or other organic source.

Likewise, asthma syndrome may start with an external trauma, including, here in New York City where we practice, from the fires of 9/11, or from the soot from thousands of diesel trucks and city buses.

As we said earlier, allergies are an immune response to proteins. Where does that put airborne pollutants?

Normally such pollutants are intercepted and expelled before they can reach the tissues. That's what the hairs in your nose, normal mucus production, cilia in the airways, and other defenses do. Heavy pollution from industrial sources, fires, or cigarettes penetrate deep into previously protected tissues, irritating sensitive airway tissues and mobilizing their defenses to get rid of the foreign matter. Sneezing and mucus production are the result. You would be hard put to distinguish these reactions from an allergic response.

However, when the particles penetrate deep into the airways and do microscopic damage to these tissues, this creates openings for allergens to do their mischief much the way a nail through your sneaker punctures your foot and creates an opening for tetanus. Tetanus germs are on your skin all the time, but they don't penetrate without that nail. Heavy air pollution in one concerted exposure, as well as chronic low-level irritation, can damage the lungs to the point where true allergic asthma can take hold. The mast cells and others deep in the airways, having once been exposed, will become sensitized to certain allergens. This is the state of twitchiness that we mentioned earlier.

We like to look at it terms of rapidly reversible conditions, slowly reversible conditions, and permanent conditions. Wheezing and coughing are usually rapidly reversible, inflammation is slowly reversible, but COPD (chronic obstructive pulmonary disease), caused by emphysema for example, is permanent. We can relieve the wheezing, coughing, and inflammation, but emphysema is a fixed, permanent, irreversible disease. A recent spate of advertising for Advair may well complicate the discussion. It may suggest that by treating bronchoconstriction and inflammation we can treat COPD. Advair or Symbicort may make it easier to breathe, but they cannot control or reverse the tissue destruction from the underlying disease.

A Few Words About the Future

Distinguishing a syndrome from a disease is useful for understanding the frontiers of research into asthma. The key to an eventual cure may come only when we understand the behavior of lung tissue at the molecular level. This lies far in the future, although some work now being done is starting to hint at it, as with the cutting edge tests marketed as ImmunoCAP (see chapter 7).

Our current pharmaceutical arsenal can keep symptoms under control and prevent them from escalating into a potentially life-threatening event. Just as important is the menu of behaviors that keep these pharmaceuticals from coming into play. It's nice to know your town has a competent fire department, but that doesn't mean you can neglect the wiring in your house. Peak flow monitoring, warm-ups before exercise on cold days, treating a runny nose early, taking your controller medications—these should be seond nature. Rescue medications should be for emergencies, not for control. Likewise, control medications should not be used at their maximal levels, but as needed. Behavior is the key to minimizing the need for control. While it may some day be possible to "fix" our bodies so that they can stop doing these destructive things to themselves, in the short run, we owe it to ourselves to stop provoking our immune systems to attack.

CHAPTER 4

The Nose Knows: Upper Airway Congestion and Asthma

YOU KNOW THE OLD EXPRESSION, "KEEP YOUR NOSE CLEAN"? It means "Stay out of trouble." But to allergists, it means something else entirely. For one thing, we don't think of the nose as that thing on your face, but the network of caves and crevices that we can't see: What we might call the "greater nose," these upper airways perform a vital function for the lungs— the lower airways—in preventing the onset of an asthma attack, and therefore they should be treated with respect. Once allergic or infectious disease gets past the upper airways, they much harder to treat.

The "Other" Functions of the Nose

The nose is more than an air portal. It is also a filter, a radiator, and a humidifier. The nose and the communicating sinuses— *when clear* and thus functioning normally—process the air you breathe so that by the time it reaches asthma territory—the lungs—it is sufficiently clean, warm, and wet to penetrate into the increasingly tiny airways where the vital business of exchanging blood oxygen for carbon dioxide can take place.

This role has long been recognized at least implicitly by certain cultures, although not necessarily by doctors to the extent that it should. If you've ever taken a yoga class, where you spend a lot of time breathing air near the dusty floor of a room, you have heard the teachers instruct you to inhale and exhale through your nose instead of through your mouth, which is conventional with most exercise, possibly reflecting some ancient wisdom about the nose's importance as a filter.

These critical "other" functions of the nose are very important to understanding the overall performance of the airways.

Allergic Rhinitis and Other Nasal Problems

Rhinitis is the medical name for the things that keep your nose from operating the way it is supposed to, blocking the flow of air to the lungs. It is everywhere: By some estimates, 80 million Americans suffer from it, and half of those have allergic rhinitis. Those allergies are estimated to account for more than 800,000 missed workdays and another 800,000 days of school absence. The social and economic costs are astronomical.

How do we tell allergic rhinitis from other forms? The distinction is pretty clear cut. Allergic rhinitis has two phases. In the first, short-term mediators such as histamine and rapidly synthesized leukotrienes and prostaglandins cause itching, sneezing, runny nose, and congestion. In the second, many of these same symptoms are renewed along with an increased sensitivity to allergens, which doctors call *priming*.

These symptoms of allergic rhinitis do not overlap particularly with nonallergic rhinitis, although there is congestion in both. But forget all that—the primary difference between allergic and nonallergic rhinitis for your purposes as parents is that the allergic variety is a condition of childhood that begins to taper off in adolescence and is pretty much gone by the age of 20 in males. But that's no reason to be complacent. As you will see below in the section "One Airway, One Disease," no parent should content herself with the attitude "this too shall pass" as the child sniffs and sneezes. To the extent that this childhood condition contributes to asthma, and airway remodeling, its detrimental effects can be permanent.

We Who Are About to Sneeze Salute You

One way to tell if your child is about to have an allergic rhinitis attack is what we call the "allergic salute." Your child will begin to twitch his nose like a rabbit and then either rub the tip with a finger or rub upward with the palm of the hand. Ask your child if he knows the joke that begins, "Why is your hair green?" That was a joke created when someone watched a kid with allergic rhinitis perform the salute.

Other physical signs of allergic rhinitis are a darkening of the skin under the eyes—"allergic shiners"—and mouth breathing with an open gaping mouth. These symptoms provoke teasing from classmates.

The nose is really the gateway to the sinuses. The ethmoid (between the eye and nose), maxillary (below the eye) and frontal (above the eye) sinuses all drain their mucus in a groove below the middle turbinate, one of three turbinates or bumps on each side of the nose.

When rhinitis or other congestion is accompanied by poor sinus drainage, it can be compounded by bacterial infection. The condition is called *sinusitis*. The allergic component will be treated with antihistamines and anti-inflammatories to promote drainage. The bacterial infection will probably be treated with antibiotics.

Sinusitis is a condition where the paradox of allergic inflammation applies, specifically that good inflammation—the inflammation involved in fighting bacterial infection—will be suppressed if steroids are used to treat allergic inflammation. The use of steroids will prolong the bacterial inflammation, yet it may be absolutely necessary if it means controlling asthma.

How Crooked Is Crooked

We all have a partially bony septum dividing the two halves of our nose. Because each half of our body does not perfectly match the other half, we often have what is called a crooked septum. But is it crooked enough to block the drainage of the sinuses? In our opinion, most times it is not crooked enough to warrant traditional surgery. We would first recommend an endoscopic look at the sinus drainage under the middle turbinate. Sometimes a simple repair of the opening with a surgical endoscope will do.

Down the Eustachian Tubes

Centuries ago, European court painters depicted children as small adults. We now know that this is the case neither anatomically, nor psychologically, nor intellectually. What does this have to do with allergy?

Look at a newborn baby's head size. It is 25 percent of the infant's body size. An adult's head size is about 12 to 15 percent of the body. Contrary to what some of our children think, this does not mean we get dumber as we get older. It means that as we get older, certain pieces of our upper airways change their relationship to one another, and that can lead to changes in our health.

The bit of anatomy we are particularly concerned with is the *Eustachian tube*, which runs from the normally air-filled middle ear to the side and back of the mouth and throat. The throat end of this tube is C-shaped cartilage, which is closed while at rest and then opened by the surrounding muscles. As a child grows, the Eustachian tube changes its relationship to the surrounding muscles, with the result that in the period between 2 and 8 years of age it is difficult to open the tube.

In the event of allergy or enlarged lymph tissue from infection, the tube will be closed for long periods of time, creating a vacuum in the middle ear, during which fluid can accumulate, followed by one of those painful ear infections. Chronic ear infections can cause hearing loss. Sometimes a tube has to be placed in the eardrum to substitute for the blocked Eustachian tube. If your child is prone to ear infection, allergy treatment is not merely useful but necessary.

One Airway, One Disease

Whatever the specific condition of the nasal passages and their susceptibility to allergic attack, current best medical practice is to view them not in isolation from the lungs but as part of the same system. This has not always been the case, and in many quarters it still is not.

Traditionally, GPs, pediatricians, and even allergists have tended to differentiate between conditions of the upper airways—the nose, the sinuses, the ears, and the network of chambers and hollows contained within the head—and the lower airways, mainly the lungs. Since diseases of the lower airways, not just asthma, but also pneumonia and others, could be life-threatening, conditions in the upper airways were relegated to the level of merely annoying—runny nose, stuffiness, and so forth. How many times have we heard a patient say, "It's just a stuffy nose," or a parent say, "His snorting is just annoying. If the noise didn't bother me, I wouldn't have brought him to a specialist and *wasted your time*."

First, let us say, you can't waste our time.

Second, and much more important, today we know how wrong we were (or at least some of us do, because many pediatricians and GPs still get it wrong) about our priorities in treating upper and lower airway disease. Because the lung conditions are seemingly "more serious" than stuffy noses, doctors have treated the lungs separately.

Even allergists make mistakes in this regard. And for their part, parents take the line of least resistance in administering prescribed treatment to their children. Let's face it, getting children to sit still while Mom shoves a tube in their nose is a pain in the neck for Mom, not to mention what it does for the child. Thus, children are frequently overtreated with strong chemicals—steroids and bronchodilators—in the lower airways when much lower-tech preventive treatments such as irrigation of the upper airways *with salt water* would stave off the need for rescue. Simple, but yucky. In fact, the problem isn't confined to children with allergies, but it also has implications for those who suffer from frequent ear infections and thus are treated with antibiotics more than they should be.

According to one study, the strongest correlation between asthma and any other risk factor is with allergic rhinitis. People with asthma

---

ONE AIRWAY, ONE DISEASE—ONE TREATMENT

Robbie is a 3-year-old with a history of asthma that was brought under good control with the use of cromolyn, the occasional use of inhaled steroids such as Pulmicort, and a beta-agonist. (See chapter 8 for fuller discussion of asthma medication.)

During the day he seemed fine, albeit tired. Nights, however, were another matter. Then, his asthma was accompanied by excessive, sometimes uncontrollable coughing, and his sleepless parents had to deal with the usual symptoms of stress and fatigue of their own. With the introduction of the nasal wash called SaltAire (a 2%–3% salt solution instead of the 0.8% found in nasal sprays), his nose cleared, and the asthma became easier to handle. His parents regained their sanity.

— *Dr. Ehrlich*

---

also have allergic rhinitis 80 percent of the time. We have a feeling that it may be even higher than that. In any case, as you will read in the chapter on medications, some of the preparations that are used to treat allergies are also used to treat asthma, although in different chemical configurations or delivery systems.

Plain as the Nose on Your Face

As Robbie's story shows, there is clear linkage between allergic conditions in the nose and in the lungs, and it's about time we learned to do something about it. It shouldn't have taken us this long. We have always appreciated the role of the nose for drainage from the rest of the cranial cavities—not only the sinuses but the ears—through the Eustachian tubes that connect the middle ears to the pharynx at the back of the nose and throat. These cavities are always collecting bacteria, dust, and pollen from the air. When foreign substances are draining properly into the nasal cavities, and then being expelled into the atmosphere or swallowed, the body's natural defenses have much of their work done for them. There's no need for the immunoglobulins to go into action.

However, when there is blockage because the mucous membranes in the sinuses or Eustachian tubes are inflamed and produce mucus, either because of infection or allergy, these foreign substances begin to accumulate and the problems are aggravated. Inflammation increases, the immune system goes into overdrive, and the infection or allergy can spread.

How does this contribute to asthma?

In two ways. First, there is the "heightened alert" status. Remember our military metaphors to describe the immune system. Mediators, to borrow some military lingo, are "scrambled" like fighter planes and reconnaissance planes in the clogged chambers of the upper airways—that is, planes take off so they can either attack or target intruders for other forces. For our purposes, this means that the mast cells and basophils begin pumping out substances that will stimulate production of the immunoglobulins with accompanying swelling and inflammation.

Some of these histamines and longer-acting leukotrienes reach the lower airways where they will look for something to attack as well. This makes the asthmatic's already "twitchy" lungs even more sensitive.

Second, there is the effect that breathing through the mouth instead of the nose has on the lungs. As we said earlier, the nose provides a service by warming and filtering the air. Studies have shown that some asthma attacks are precipitated by breathing air that is too cold or too dry for the lungs. Athletes, for example, may suffer an asthma attack when jogging on a cool day before their lower airways are sufficiently warm. But even non-athletes will suffer if their noses are stuffed up—not an unlikely event during cold season, or for allergy sufferers cooped up in school or at home with stale, dusty, hot, dry air who then emerge into freezing or near-freezing winter air.

Natural Radiator and Humidifier

You may have noticed that if you breathe rapidly, as you would when running for a bus on a very cold day, you begin to cough. This is because the cold air is causing constriction of the airways, a reflex that protects the delicate tissues deep inside the lungs. A well-functioning nose will warm that cold air. Without the humidity supplied by the nose, the lung tissues will dry out, and the mucus will thicken and become too difficult to bring out. We often describe to our patients the analogy, as unsavory as it may be, of a glob of mucus on a glass slide. Left alone or fanned, the mucus becomes dry, thick, and difficult to scrape off the slide. If it is treated with well-humidified air, the mucus is easier to scrape off.

Warming Up Before Exercise

We have a couple of suggestions regarding what to do before exercising outdoors in cool weather, one that involves medicine and equipment and one that does not.

Simply take a few laps in a warm gym before going outside. The flow of air in and out of the airways cools the lungs before they warm up again with exercise. If an asthmatic goes directly from warm inside temperatures to cold outside temperatures, the shock causes bronchospasm. It is better to gradually pre-cool the airways with an indoor warm-up so that the contrast will not be so great.

The other is to take Proventil or another beta-agonist spray twenty minutes before exercise to prevent bronchial spasms and to wear a facemask of the kind used by carpenters to trap and pre-warm air, then engage in a normal warm-up. Studies have shown that rapid cooling of the airways followed by re-warming causes coughing in some and wheezing in others. Warmed and moistened air will minimize this response, which is why asthmatics have few wheezing problems swimming in pools, where the water is continually evaporating.

Based on what we know now, we can see that the allergic activity taking place in a stuffy nose means that the lungs will be more prone to an asthma attack. The whole thing is a self-feeding, self-compounding process. In military terms, international tensions are high, and the armed forces are on alert.

They can easily escalate into the "war" of acute asthma. At that point there may be no choice but to bring in the heavy artillery and saturation bombing of bronchodilators and steroids delivered by a nebulizer—a device in which the medicine is vaporized ultrasonically or thermally and conveyed via a tube through a mask that fits over the mouth and nose.

Confusion About Allergies and Asthma

It is understandable that patients, parents, and doctors would focus on the debilitating, life-threatening asthma condition and give short shrift to the annoying, messy problem of allergic rhinitis. Pediatric training has long held that the problems could be regarded separately, and indeed many of our patients come to us from pediatricians who still say, "It's just a stuffy nose—but the asthma is a serious condition." In fact, antihistamines, which are very effective in treating allergic nasal and sinus congestion, are still largely avoided when the patient is asthmatic because they tend to dry out mucous membranes.

Doctors will tell their patients that anything that might dry out the lungs is bad for their asthma. Current research tells us something else: that histamine accounts for approximately half the symptoms characteristic of upper-airway disease. Contrary to the popular wisdom about dryness in the lungs, by limiting the allergic reaction in the upper airways the antihistamines more than counter any drying effects by allowing nature's humidifier to work the way it's supposed to.

At this point in the history of allergy treatment, the upper and lower airways cannot and should not be separated. One of our patients, hearing of the relationship of the two airways, suddenly came up with a concise analogy: "Oh, it's like a long garden hose with a nut stuck way in one end [the nose]. Ninety-nine percent of the hose may be completely functional, but that one little obstruction can cause a lot of trouble. With asthma, you recognize there's a problem at the other end [the lungs], but you have to care for where the air comes in first."

Never forget that every overt asthma attack or incidence of "silent" pre-asthma or post-asthma may take a long-term toll on vital lung function. You wouldn't want to fill the leaky radiator of your car with antifreeze every time you drive; you'd want to fix the leak. Well, neither do you want to medicate your child's asthmatic lungs with bronchodilators every time he goes outside in the winter if you can give his body's own intricate machinery a chance to do the job it's supposed to do before he runs into trouble.

Furthermore, because early-phase inflammatory mediators like histamine are present in both upper airway allergy and asthma, modern antihistamines administered in dosages that are appropriate for allergic rhinitis may help stave off subsequent asthma attacks or diminish their severity. An antihistamine like cetirizine (marketed under the brand name Zyrtec) and other so-called second-generation antihistamines such as Claritin or Allegra, may reduce the dosages required for rescue doses of the bronchodilator albuterol.

As you can see, sometimes the solution is simple, but the problem is still not easily resolved because administering the treatment itself is difficult. Very small children do not like having Mom mess with their noses. They will put up such a fight that Mom will give up and content herself to just keep up with the dosing of powerful, but convenient, medication. For her part, she is so embarrassed by the fact that she's cowed by a 2-year-old that she will fail to share this information with the allergist.

Tsk, tsk, Mom. This has happened again and again. As you will read in chapter 7, a good medical history is the most important ingredient of allergic diagnosis and treatment, and history does not end when you walk out of the allergist's office after the first visit.

An allergic medical history is ongoing. It must be updated. If your small child is resisting the prescribed treatment, tell your doctor. The only parental failure involved is when you don't do things that you should have done. Let your doctor help find a solution to the problem of administering treatment. Don't allow medication fatigue to come between your child and his or her health!

Older children don't like doing icky stuff to themselves or, for that matter, any course of treatment that requires remembering a routine. They, too, would often rather rely on the immediate gratification of bronchodilators instead of the preventive regimen of irrigating their sinuses.

A DEEPER LOOK

We had a 4-year-old patient who was using bronchodilators, inhaled steroids, and oral steroids for his asthma. I was able to look at the turbinates—several folds of tissue at the front or anterior region of the nasal passages—which were clear. However, for a deeper look into the posterior chambers, we had to sedate him. We found severe swelling of the tissue and heavy production of mucus that never managed to escape. In effect, this was a nose that was blocked but never ran.

By washing the area and applying steroids that had never been able to penetrate that deep, we were able to shrink the tissues so that his mom could irrigate him with the hypertonic saline washes and sprayed steroids on a daily basis. Over a not-very-long time, we were able to wean him from the asthma medications, and thus reduce his steroid intake almost entirely. The daily ordeal of giving several medications became a breeze when reduced to one— literally and figuratively a breath of fresh air.   — *Dr. Ehrlich*

There's an old saw: An ounce of prevention is worth a pound of cure. However, sometimes it looks the other way around: An ounce of cure in the form of a bronchodilator is preferable to a pound of time-consuming and gross prevention.

No good! The cycle of chronic asthmatic inflammation and bouts of wheezing followed by powerful quick-acting drugs is a vicious one. Those ounces of cure can add up to a ton of damage to the lungs.

Tips for a Healthy Nose—and Lungs

Know your medications! Antihistamines like fexofenadine (prescription Allegra), loratadine (off prescription Claritin), and cetirizine (off prescription Zyrtec), or levocetirizine dihydrochloride, a refined version of cetirizine (prescription Xyzal) help cut down on sneezing and dry up runny noses, but do not relieve congestion. For that you need decongestants such as pseudoephedrine.

Prescription corticosteroid nasal sprays such as Nasonex, Rhinocort, or Nasacort can help with all symptoms. Desloratadine (sold as Clarinex) is said to have some decongestant activity, but this medication is not recommended for children under the age of 12.

Keep your nose wet! Wet nasal passages do everything they're supposed to do better than dry ones. We recommend that you irrigate your nasal passages with saline solutions with high concentrations of salt, 2%–3%, because the salt draws moisture into the mucous membranes from surrounding tissues by osmosis, thus hastening the restoration of the membranes' natural irrigating function. We were given the recipe for this hypertonic salt solution by two ENT (ear, nose, and throat) specialists and is as follows: one quart of tap water, two to three heaping teaspoons of sea salt or kosher salt (both have no additives), and one level teaspoon of baking soda (such as Arm & Hammer).

Marketed as SaltAire and Ocean among other names, saline solutions come ready-made in a plastic squeeze bottle for easy inhalation of the solution. You may buy a similar bottle or purchase a 30 cc bulb syringe for administering your own low-cost home brew.

Don't let your teenager go overboard on over-the-counter nasal sprays! Too much of a good thing can hurt the patient. A medication like oxymetazoline hydrochloride, marketed as Afrin or Neo-Synephrine—once available by prescription, but now available without—provides profound relief as swollen blood vessels in the nasal passages shrink, restricting the painful flow of fluids into the nose and sinuses. But when the effect wears off it makes the patient feel miserable. The vessels dilate to more than their previous diameter, literally becoming engorged; the congestion increases. Thus, these sprays require further use for relief.

Long-term repetition of this cycle makes the nasal blood vessels and tissues look like raw hamburger and is called *rhinitis medicamentosa*, or "inflammation of the nose secondary to medication." This is not a problem for every child, but it is for teenagers who don't want to talk to their parents about their problems, let alone have Mom or Dad send them to the pediatrician, so they will go to the drugstore and buy a cheap generic version of this stuff. Unlike other over-the-counter medicines that are abused by teens, there's no euphoria. They don't get high. But the absence of discomfort alone is exhilarating enough for some. According to our local pharmacists, the stuff flies off the shelves. It shouldn't. (More discussion in chapter 8.)

Tell your allergist about all other medications your teenager is using! With adult patients, medications unrelated to allergy can exacerbate allergic problems. For example, blood pressure medicines can cause nasal congestion. So can birth control pills. Your teenage daughter may be on birth control pills, if not for contraceptive purposes then for regulating her periods or for her skin. Tell your allergist about any such drugs!

Irrigate when you fly! The very low humidity on airplanes combined with changes in cabin pressure can wreak havoc on tear ducts and sinuses, both of which play a role in staving off allergic attacks. Moreover, there's the danger of exposure to airborne germs as air recirculates. Protect your child's defenses with regular saline irrigation before you take off and while aloft. Make him drink plenty of liquids, too.

Keep nasal sprays away from the middle of the nose! This area, which is comprised of bone and cartilage, is prone to nosebleeds from exposure to medications. Regular reliance on nasal sprays may give your teenager the appearance of being a chronic cocaine user.

Intranasal Steroids (INS), Cleared for Use by Young Children

Since we wrote the first version of this book, a very effective class of medications has been cleared for use by young children. Intranasal steroids were formerly only recommended for those above the age of 12. Like all local steroids, such as inhaled or topical ones, targeted application avoids the general effects that make systemic corticosteroids so problematic for the immune system as a whole. The most prominent of the intranasal steroids is made with a drug called ciclesonide, which is currently being heavily promoted as Omnaris.

As with inhaled steroids, INS aren't used for emergencies. When a child needs to decongest, there's no substitute for the kinds of treatment described above. However, by controlling inflammation, in this case in the nasal passages and sinuses, INS can be very helpful in getting ready for predictable events like the advent of pollen season, when you know your child's nose is going to explode, clog up, or both. Premedication with INS and an antihistamine approximately two weeks before the start of the season is usually very helpful, and continuing that care for the balance will make a big difference. Different drugs are recommended for different age groups, such as mometasone furoate monohydrate, sold as Nasonex, and triamcinolone acetonide, sold as Nasacort.

CHAPTER 5

Food, Glorious Food?

POP QUIZ

How many Americans have food allergies?

A. 2 percent

B. 13–18 percent

How many Americans *think* they have food allergies?

A. 2 percent

B. 13–18 percent

YEARS AGO WHEN DR. CHIARAMONTE, ONE OF YOUR AUTHORS, helped conduct a survey about perceptions of food allergy, the answers were 2 percent and 13–18 percent, respectively. The numbers were comparable in European countries, so this was not just a question of nutty, neurotic Americans imagining there is something wrong with them.

Today, the numbers have risen. According to the World Allergy Organization, 4 percent of adults and 6 percent of children under the age of 3 have food allergy. This results in 125,000 emergency room visits each year. However, now, as in the days when this survey was carried out, many more people think they have food allergies than actually have them. If anything, more problems are probably attributed to food allergies than ever before; we therefore feel very strongly that the reality of these allergies be clearly understood.

Food allergies differ from other allergies because even a minuscule amount of the wrong food can be fatal, whereas the severity of other allergic attacks is usually proportional to the size of the dose. Traces of the offending food in poorly labeled processed foods, on cross-contaminated utensils, and carried on the hands of others pose a constant threat to those with food allergies.

There are people who will never go to a baseball game because someone nearby might buy peanuts and Cracker Jacks. Moreover, there are no national guidelines on food preparation for manufacturers, and the labeling of ingredients, although regulated, is misleading almost by design.

The only true treatment for an episode of anaphylaxis is an injection of epinephrine, a synthetic version of the body's own adrenaline. It works by stimulating the release of both beta-1 and beta-2 neurotransmitters, and thus is known as a *beta-agonist*.

Beta-1 neurotransmitters constrict the blood vessels and increase the tone of the veins, raising blood pressure, which is desirable because of loss of fluid from the blood during anaphylaxis. Not only are vital organs deprived of oxygen when blood pressure goes down, but the

---

THE DRUNKEN FIREFIGHTER

Ray was a fireman, a big strong guy whose job was to go in first and carry out people who were unconscious or trapped. At one fire Ray had rescued a 4-year-old girl from certain death. Elated with the rescue, Ray happily grabbed a coffee and donut from an onlooker who had shown up to support the brave crew. Suddenly, strapping Ray who had braved the fire unharmed and robust was faint. His captain looked at him and asked, "Ray, have you been drinking?" —surely an insult to a man who routinely risked his life.

In fact, Ray's throat was closing. He looked at the donut. It had peanuts on it. He held up his Medic Alert bracelet, which identified him as allergic to peanuts, and gave his EpiPen (an injectable-epinephrine device) to the captain just before he collapsed. The captain, who of course had been trained in first aid, gave him the injection. A piece of peanut almost accomplished what years of fighting fires never did: kill Ray.   — *Dr. Chairamonte*

---

blood vessels themselves leak, much in the way the joints in your hot water pipes will leak if the pump fails because they depend on pressure to keep all the seals tight.

Beta-2 relaxes the smooth bronchial muscles and opens up constricted airways, which allows the patient suffering from anaphylactic shock to breathe. An epinephrine dose lasts twenty to thirty minutes after which the patient may require another injection as well as oral or intravenous fluids to expand the blood volume.

Epinephrine is a very powerful drug. Like adrenaline, it provides you with an extra jolt of strength and energy in an emergency, the so-called fight-or-flight response. The stimulation it provides to the heart can be frightening to a child, particularly when the child is already disturbed because of anaphylaxis. As we mentioned in chapter 4, asthmatics commonly use another beta-agonist, albuterol, which only works with beta-2 and leaves the heart alone. Because of this, it is much more suitable for regular use as a rescue medication for asthma, although it's not without problems.

With epinephrine, as with albuterol, the best use of the medication is to manage the condition so that rescue is never required. (By the way, while this is not terribly relevant for children, those who are treated for high blood pressure and other conditions with drugs called beta-blockers should avoid epinephrine and other beta-agonists since their actions negate one another.)

Each year, some 2,000 Americans are hospitalized, and 200 die, from eating foods that for the vast majority of people are nutritious and perfectly safe.

Outgrowth

The incidence of food allergy is much higher for children than for adults: 8 percent of those under three, and rising. The reason for the much higher rate among kids is partly the result of the fact that most people "outgrow" their food allergies, peanuts being the exception. Only 10 to 20 percent lose their peanut allergy as opposed to 90 percent for other foods. Milk allergy is often the result of an immature digestive system that can't handle the complex proteins at an early age, but that eventually does mature.

However, the fact that the numbers of food-allergic children are growing may well indicate that there are other things at work that are compromising the way their immune systems are developing. As we said in an earlier chapter, the first social change that may have given rise to allergy was the invention of the shoe, which kept parasites from entering children's feet. Then it was energy-efficient housing. Now it may well be that the almost universal use of antibiotics in young children has subverted the immune system from fighting germs to reacting to foods and other allergens in an allergic fashion. T-helper lymphocyte cells are redirecting the B-lymphocyte cells that produce all the different kinds of antibodies from making the germ-fighting IgG to the allergic antibody IgE. With fewer germs to fight, the T cells start pushing the B cells to make more IgE.

Passing It On

Heredity may cause a predisposition to allergies of any type, including food allergy, but so may prenatal care: Several studies have indicated that mothers who breast-feed their babies and avoid major food allergens may deter the subsequent development of some food allergies in their children.

Most patients who have true food allergies have other types of allergies as well, such as dust or pollen, and children with both food allergies and asthma are at increased risk for more severe reactions.

Proteins—Building Blocks and Stumbling Blocks of Life

Proteins ... can't live without them, can't live with them. When we develop sensitivity to food or dust or pollens, we are really developing sensitivity to the proteins in them. Don't forget that our allergic reactions are really leftover immune responses to parasites, and parasites are worms, not-so-simple protein-rich life forms. When these new allergens enter our system in the form of unfamiliar, complex protein, the immune system goes into action. Thus, some of the proteins in cow's milk may look to a North American immune system like some diarrhea-inducing bug still found on the Nile. Or something in egg whites might look like something lying dormant in an old potato field in Poland.

Egg whites are pure protein, as opposed to the yolk that feeds on the white during the gestation of a chicken. But the same thing that makes egg white so attractive to diet-conscious adults—thus the popularity of egg white omelets—makes it problematic for children with allergic tendencies.

We can't live without proteins. They are the building blocks of life, as every ninth-grade biology student learns. They are the stuff that muscle is made of.

Until her first birthday, however, a child's gut may not be able to break the proteins down into their constituent amino acids, the building blocks of protein, which are too small to cause allergy. When these undigested proteins build up, they are treated like any other allergens. The immune system goes into action, producing IgE. Normally, there is IgA immunoglobulin present to protect against IgE production. However, for some babies, IgA production is delayed, and IgE does its destructive work.

One child in 200 has no IgA. Their digestive systems are overwhelmed by milk. The equivalent of a 10-pound baby drinking one quart of milk a day would be a 150-pound adult drinking fifteen quarts, or nearly four gallons, per day.

In these instances, when the child is unable to handle these complex proteins, we have to look for alternatives that they can digest. This is a search for simplicity. The next step is to find simpler proteins, such as the vegetable proteins in soy. They have enough protein to use as cattle feed but are simple enough for a cow's vegetarian digestive system. However, for the one-third of milk-allergic infants who become allergic to soy, the alternatives must be simpler still.

The most allergy-neutral form of protein one can eat is not the building blocks of life themselves but the building blocks of the building blocks—amino acids. And that is the premise of such new products as EleCare, which contains such amino acids as lysine, leucine, and glutamine, along with corn syrup solids, oils, and vitamin and mineral supplements. The amino acids are ingested as separate components of protein and then assembled inside the digestive tract.

However, each layer of new, more scientifically advanced food carries an escalating price tag. Better to stave off each new level of allergic sensitivity in the first place with measures like careful diet for food allergy as well as better housekeeping, filtering the air that the child sleeps in, and, in many heartrending cases, getting rid of pets for other allergies.

Food Allergies—Real Problems Whatever the Origins

Whatever the reasons our children have their food allergies, the problem is very real. No one knows this better than Anne Muñoz-Furlong, who founded the Food Allergy & Anaphylaxis Network (FAAN) out of her frustration while trying to solve the problem of her child's milk allergy. For many months she was told by a succession of doctors that her daughter (whose symptoms were poor sleep, projectile vomiting immediately after being fed, severe cramping, and endless bouts of painful eczema starting at the age of 9 months) was too young to be allergic, that she was just a fussy baby, and that Anne herself was a fussy mother. It took many months and the family being told to avoid a variety of foods before they were referred to an allergist.

"It would have been easier if the condition were life threatening," says Anne. "Then my daughter would have been seen by doctors who would have made the diagnosis right away."

Anne's trial-and-error odyssey to specialist treatment was painful for the whole family. Her older, nonallergic daughter was like a "forgotten child," so consuming were the problems of the younger one. The difficult experience was the basis of her starting a newsletter to help other parents, and out of that, the FAAN was born.

Anaphylaxis—Nothing But the Facts

The greatest danger from food allergy is anaphylaxis, also known as anaphylactic shock, a violent allergic reaction involving a number of parts of the body simultaneously.

Like less serious reactions, anaphylaxis usually occurs after a person has already been exposed to an allergen, although it can appear to happen the first time a person eats a particular food. Any food can trigger anaphylaxis but the basic list is short.

The Basic Food Allergy Groups

While any food can cause allergies, 90 percent of all food-allergic reactions are caused by:

- **Milk** (number one food allergen for those under age of 3 years)
- **Peanuts** (number one food allergen for those over age of 3 years), which are not really nuts at all, but legumes
- **Eggs**
- **Shellfish**
- **Fish**
- **Soy**
- **Wheat**
- **Tree nuts,** such as walnuts and pecans, which are nuts.

UNJUST DESSERT

Halfway through my pie, my mouth began to itch and I told my mother that I was afraid the pie must have contained peanuts. Having lived through this before, my parents and I began to feel a sense of impending doom. On the other hand, we guessed that if there had been any peanuts in the pie, the amount must have been minuscule, and we knew that my medicine was close at hand, so we decided to sit tight and wait it out.

Over the next five minutes the itching in my mouth became more intense but I otherwise felt okay. My parents decided it would be best to give me a dose of Benadryl. They were confident it would be enough.

Shortly thereafter, I noticed that my palms and soles were becoming itchy and felt that my lips were slightly swollen. I sat quietly and waited for the Benadryl to work.

A minute or two later my mother noted that my face was flushed and my lips were swollen. Within ten minutes I was covered with hives, had swelling of my eyes and lips, and was beginning to wheeze. I used my EpiPen and we left for the hospital. On the way there I experienced more and more trouble breathing. I felt like my chest was tight and that my throat was starting to close off. I itched all over and felt a little light-headed.

— *Thirteen-year-old boy,*
Stories from the Heart:
A Collection of Essays from Teens with Food Allergies

As little as one-fifth to one five-thousandth of a teaspoon of the offending food has proved fatal.

A small amount of the offending protein is absorbed essentially intact into the body, bypassing the digestive process. The protein combines with at least two allergic IgE antibodies attached to a mast cell. The antibody has been made from a prior exposure to the protein—this is, after all, an amnesic or remembered response. They fit with the allergic food protein like a key into a lock.

This union of the food protein and two bound IgE antibodies activates the mast cell to release chemicals that are the cause of the allergic reaction and all the armed forces come into play, like histamine, leukotrienes, and prostaglandins, and eosinophils, neutrophils, and platelets.

With all these agents activated, epinephrine must be given early to call off the red alert and the catastrophe of anaphylaxis.

Anaphylaxis can produce severe symptoms in as little as five to fifteen minutes, although life-threatening reactions may progress over hours.

Signs of such a reaction include: difficulty breathing, feeling of impending doom, swelling of the mouth and throat, a drop in blood pressure, and loss of consciousness. The sooner anaphylaxis is treated, the greater the chance of surviving. The episode should involve a trip to the emergency room, even if symptoms seem to subside on their own

Hope for Peanut Allergy Sufferers? Not Yet

Sometimes medical science outruns economics, and some-times it's the other way around. An experimental drug called TNX-901 was announced in 2003. When injected once a month, it was supposed to protect peanut allergy sufferers from inadvertent ingestion of the dreaded legume. However, the company that developed it was acquired by a bigger company and it was discontinued.

Living with Food Allergy

There is no specific test to predict the likelihood of anaphylaxis, although testing may provide some guidance as to the severity of the allergy. Experts advise those who are susceptible to anaphylaxis to carry medication, such as injectable epinephrine, at all times, and to check the medicine's expiration date regularly.

Doctors can instruct patients with allergies on how to self-administer epinephrine. Prompt treatment can be a life-or-death matter. Injectable epinephrine is a synthetic version of the natural hormone adrenaline. For treatment of an anaphylactic reaction, it is injected directly into a thigh muscle and works directly on the cardiovascular and respiratory systems, causing rapid constriction of blood vessels, reversing throat swelling, relaxing lung muscles to improve breathing, and stimulating the heartbeat.

Epinephrine for emergency home use comes in three forms: a traditional needle and syringe kit known as Ana-Kit, an auto

---

GENETICALLY MODIFIED PEANUTS?

One of the more intriguing factoids in our field is that in all of China, which has four times the U.S. population, the number of people with peanut allergies is the same. Can it be something in the peanuts? One theory is that American companies are modifying the peanuts genetically. There is no question that genetic modification constitutes a threat. A Japanese-American consortium had genetically produced lysergic acid, the same compound in warm milk and turkey that makes us sleepy, as a "natural sleeping pill." Some trace by-product of the pill managed to kill several hundred Americans before the Japanese withdrew it and hid the production records from the FDA. This precedent proves there's ample reason to worry, but how worried is another matter. One trouble is that the Food and Drug Administration is better at regulating drugs than food. As long as a new food is substantially the same as an old one, it doesn't need exhaustive study for use. But altering the chemistry of food can produce a compound as powerful as a new drug. For now, there's no 100 percent certainty, so read labels carefully, and cook with care.

By the way, there have been efforts to genetically modify peanuts without the offending proteins, but by all accounts, the result tastes awful. — *Dr. Chairamonte*

---

matic injector system known as EpiPen, and the more recent Twin-ject. EpiPen's automatic injector design, which was originally developed for use by military personnel to deliver nerve gas antidotes, is described by some as a "fat pen." The patient removes the safety cap and pushes the automatic injector tip against the outer thigh until the unit activates. The patient holds the "pen" in place for several seconds, then throws it away. While an EpiPen delivers one pre-measured dosage, the Ana-Kit provides two doses, which makes it unnecessary to carry a back-up. A second dose may be required in up to 20 percent of reactions, ten to fifteen minutes after the first dose.

The newer device, Twinject, appeals to pediatric allergists for three reasons: (1) the bore of the needle is narrower and less painful to our little patients (or to big ones for that matter); (2) the epinephrine is injected with a much "softer" shot, with an injection pressure of 6 pounds per square inch (compared to EpiPen's 30 psi), making it somewhat more kid friendly; and (3) it has a second dose "behind" the first. It's also a smaller instrument and therefore easier to carry.

The injectable-epinephrine industry is a case study in the functioning of the market in health care delivery, with both positive and negative implications. It's also an affirmation of our decision to create a web complement to our book, because things happen very rapidly. In the past month during production of this book, both Twinject (now owned by a new company) and EpiPen have launched new products in response to competition with one another. For its part, when people complained that the second dose might be given by accident, the new Twinject company came out with a single-dose device. The EpiPen company came out with a needle-safety apparatus, although it is not without its problems. One critical element that the manufacturers—and their doctors— should keep in mind is that treatment for anaphylaxis is usually self-treatment. Our patients and their families have used one system for years. Changing their behavior to accommodate new technology will entail unlearning the old and learning the new. In an emergency—and using injectable epinephrine is always an emergency—means remembering to do it the new way. Doctors, parents, kids, school nurses, babysitters: Learn the new way of doing things before you need it!

For further developments, follow us on AsthmaAllergiesChildren. com.

Advice from Study

Hugh A. Sampson, MD, the foremost food allergy expert, and his erstwhile colleagues at Baltmore's Johns Hopkins (he is now at Mount Sinai), published a study of anaphylactic reactions in children in the *New England Journal of Medicine* (Aug. 6, 1992) involving thirteen children who had severe allergic reactions to food. Six died, and seven nearly died.

Among the study's conclusions:

• Asthma, a disease with allergic underpinnings, was common to all children in the study.

• Epinephrine should be prescribed and kept available for those with severe food allergies.

• Children who have an allergic reaction should be observed for three to four hours after a reaction in a medical center capable of dealing with anaphylaxis.

• Timing is crucial. The shorter the time that lapses between ingesting the offending food and taking the epinephrine, the better the chance of survival.

Eternal Vigilance

Anne Muñoz-Furlong points out that there is a steep learning curve for any food allergy family. "Parents come to us in a state of disbelief. They give their children something that is 'good' for them and end up in an emergency room. The doctors tell them it is life-threatening. Suddenly a perfectly normal child in every other respect has a sword of Damocles hanging over their head, and so does the family." After their own stage of "grief," there's disbelief, then acceptance, and then they have the problem of convincing everyone else that it's real. People look at them as though they're claiming to have been abducted by aliens.

They know that the price of a healthy child is eternal vigilance, and even then things can go wrong. Anne tells of one family where a mother was chatting happily with her milk-allergic daughter. She poured herself a glass of milk while her daughter poured some soy milk for herself. There was a mix-up. "One minute they were chatting about going to the mall, and the next, the mother was calling 911."

Misunderstanding Food Allergy

The incidence of food allergy is on the rise, but so is the consciousness of it and with that comes a big increase in self-diagnosis, sometimes right and sometimes wrong, and treatment, right or wrong. But it is also wildly misunderstood, so all kinds of symptoms are attributed to food allergy that have nothing to do with it. The misinformation and misconceptions that have sprung up around it distract from wider understanding of the severity of the real thing.

Some of the misunderstanding results from confusion of food allergy with other real but nevertheless nonallergic ailments. The best example of this is lactose intolerance. A child, or an adult for that matter, may not be able to tolerate milk and have severe diarrhea or vomiting, but when examined more closely it is discovered that he cannot digest the foods, not that he is allergic.

"THEY" DON'T UNDERSTAND

On June 10, 2001, I was quoted in the *New York Times Magazine* as saying: I tell my patients, if people point at you when you walk down the street and say, "Look at that neurotic parent," then and only then are you being careful enough.

I said it, and I meant it, but upon reflection, it bears further explanation. By "neurotic" I meant a selfless dedication that to outsiders could appear excessive. "They" don't understand the threat to your child. You do.

One parent quoted in the article said, "After my son was rushed to the doctor because he touched an egg noodle—just touched it—my friends finally apologized to me for what they'd been saying behind my back."

"They" don't understand what life is like … endlessly reading food packages for dangerous ingredients, never knowing whether something is not on the label, wondering when you enter a restaurant if the kitchen is well run or subtly contaminated.

For the parent of a severely food-allergic child, the world is full of hidden dangers. Food companies and their lapdogs in government look more conspiratorial than the CIA in an Oliver Stone movie. The regulations and the bureaucracies growing up to cope with the problems are daunting, frustrating, and sometimes contradictory.

You can't be too careful. There used to be a saying, "Just because you're paranoid doesn't mean those people *aren't looking at you.*" At the same time, reality is hard enough. Food allergy turns childhood into a time of *Alice in Wonderland* logic. Up is down and black is white. Don't let it reach the point of unreality.　— *Dr. Ehrlich*

Flour Power—The Gluten Controversy

Gluten is a real food villain. In some people it causes inflammatory changes in the gut stemming from immunological processes, although they are not related to IgE. However, the range of claims that are made about its widespread presence seems to us to be excessive. If you suspect you have a problem with gluten, eliminate it in all forms from your diet for two to four weeks and see if you feel better.

There is such a thing as "baker's asthma." That is asthma prompted by inhaling some—not all—flours. The reaction is to inhaling airborne flour, not to handling or ingesting dough. We have found positive IgE-mediated skin tests in some cases but not in others.

A Texas woman found a silver lining: Because of the wide availability of Mexican food, which is based on corn, gluten-sensitive people don't have as big a problem there as those in other parts of the country.

Guide to the Worry Years

In the first year of a child's life, a parent has almost total control over the child. Between one and two, the child starts to "cruise," i.e., get around the house, so anything within range of the child's hand is also within range of her mouth. Since there is no reasoning with a child that age, the responsibility for making sure that nothing allergenic is within reach.

When the "terrible twos" begin, you can communicate with the child, but she will be oppositional; she will hear what you tell her to do and not do, and do the opposite. After about two and a half, a child will begin to pay attention and can begin to participate in policing her own behavior. As she acquires words, things like milk, eggs, and peanuts can be associated with the substances themselves. In a couple of years, she can begin to read labels on her own. This spirit of cooperation lasts until the teenage years, when behavior and knowledge part ways again.

THE LONELINESS OF THE PARENT OF THE FOOD-ALLERGIC CHILD

We've been greatly hurt by some people's reactions: "Why don't you just home school?" "It's not our problem." "Aren't you making a big deal out of nothing?" "How serious can it be?" "What harm can just a little bit do?" "I think you're just being overprotective." "You must have eaten something you shouldn't have when you were pregnant." "We'd love to baby-sit for you, but it would be too scary." "Hasn't he outgrown this yet?" "We'd have invited you to the party, but we didn't want to change the menu." It is sad to learn how many would rather have an egg breakfast than our company—we're much more fun than eggs, we really are.

— *Kathy Lundquist,*
Stories from Parents' Hearts:
Essays by Parents of Children with Food Allergies

School Food and Allergies by the Numbers

Nearly two-thirds of all school districts (65.3 percent) have not banned any foods due to food allergies. Only about one in ten districts have banned certain foods in all of their schools; an additional 22 percent have done so in some schools. Peanuts are the most commonly banned food item, with nearly 96 percent of districts with a food ban in place targeting the ban of peanuts. (Statistics are from "State of School Nutrition 2009," which can be found at www.schoolnutrition.org.)

For the record, we agree with the Food Allergy & Anaphylaxis Network that foods *should **not** be banned* from school. Their reasoning is twofold: One is that it's not the real world. The second is that many schools convince the parents that they are peanut (or other foods) free. Allergen-sensitive children and their parents gain a false sense of security and let down their guard. There is also the fact that kids cheat.

SCIENCE OR NO SCIENCE?

For over twenty years I have been involved in fending off disinformation about food allergy. For the record, food allergy is an immune response to certain foods. It is not a catchall for vague complaints about mood or energy levels or behavior. Nor is it the cause of a perceived increase in ADHD, autism, or even asthma, which is the current line of discussion.

It's hard enough to get good medical science into common use. When it's arrayed against the false medicine that people want to believe, it's much more difficult. Whenever this happens, I think of the words of that eminent Italian American philosopher Yogi Berra: "It's déjà vu all over again." The situation is complicated by the fact that there are elements of each that are implicated in all the others. For example, sleep disturbance from allergy and asthma presents itself in the inattentiveness and bad behavior that is sometimes treated as ADHD. Autistic children may be intolerant of certain foods, but food intolerance is not allergy. Many people who traffic in disinformation are quite well meaning, and desperate to find hope in an apparently hopeless cause. But others, like the Russians who coined the word *disinformation* in 1955, have an agenda, like selling false cures, or even books.

Real food allergy manifests itself very shortly after ingesting the offending foods in a limited number of distinct ways.

— *Dr. Chiaramonte*

Foods and Asthma

Asthma from food allergy is relatively uncommon. Food allergies affect less than 1 percent of adults, and up to 5 percent of children. Asthmatics are more likely than non-asthmatics to experience severe allergic reactions to foods, and asthmatics have a higher risk of death if they experience food anaphylaxis.

Allergy and Intolerance—Different Problems

The difference between an allergy and an intolerance is how the body handles the offending food; that is, whether the reaction involves the immune system or not. With a true food allergy, the body's immune system recognizes an allergen as foreign and produces antibodies to halt the "invasion." The most common battlefields are the mouth (swelling of the lips), digestive tract (stomach cramps, vomiting, diarrhea), skin (hives, rashes, or eczema), and the airways (wheezing or breathing).

Food intolerance is much more common than allergy. The problem is not with the body's immune system, but rather with its ability to process certain compounds—hence the diarrhea and vomiting with lactose intolerance. Patients are usually deficient in the intestinal enzyme lactase, which is needed to digest milk sugar. Estimates are that about 80 percent of African Americans have lactose intolerance, as do many people of Mediterranean or Hispanic origin.

Intolerance has also been reported over the years to certain food additives, including aspartame, a sweetener; monosodium glutamate (MSG), a flavor enhancer; sulfur-based preservatives; and tartrazine, also known as FD&C Yellow No. 5, a food color.

Again, these are not allergies.

PSEUDO FOOD ALLERGY

Food and the rituals of mealtime are an important glue that holds families and households together, which is healthy when families are healthy but can be part of a family problem if the family is troubled. When I see a patient who claims to be allergic to twenty foods or more, and their symptoms are vague and variable and don't appear for more than twelve hours after eating, I start to ask if there's anything unusual going on at home because I suspect that the "allergies" are part of some other problem.

Sometimes the extent to which people will go to deal with their imagined allergies is astonishing. Years ago, I was skin testing a young woman named Alice in connection to her very real asthma. I noticed some strange lumps around her joints and asked her to see a rheumatologist. He examined her and informed me that she had scurvy—a disease resulting from vitamin C deficiency that used to afflict sailors on long sea voyages hundreds of years ago—something that present-day doctors almost never see. Hundreds of *(continued on next page)*

---

years ago, the Royal Navy figured out that scurvy could be prevented by consumption of fresh limes—hence the word "limey," which the English are known as to this day. Alice managed to contract scurvy because of the "anti-allergic" diet she contrived for herself for her self-diagnosed allergies. She thought that she was allergic to corn and corn products like corn syrup among many other foods. Try reading labels and see how many things have corn products in them. But her diet must also have excluded fresh uncooked fruit and vegetables of all kinds, since most of them contain traces of vitamin C.

I sent her to Johns Hopkins for food challenge studies in which potential problem foods are given in a controlled setting so that a bad reaction can be treated. I was just learning how to do them at that time. Her tests were negative but she wouldn't accept the results. She left the hospital rather than try eating corn in a protected environment. What was wrong with her? Well, the fact that her problems coincided with her breakup with a long-term boyfriend might have had something to do with it. And the fact that she was referred to me by her beautiful sister, who had always overshadowed her and was getting married, probably didn't help. I could treat her for her asthma, but not her "food allergies." And certainly not for her own very real problems.
— *Dr. Chiaramonte*

Got Milk Allergy?

True milk allergy involves the presence of an IgE antibody to one or more proteins in milk. Milk, of course, is the chief staple of infant diets, and thinking your way around milk is a real pain.

The problem arises when large amounts of intact milk proteins are absorbed through the immature gut where they present themselves to an immature immune system. At that point they stimulate an allergic response, provoking reactions ranging from mild itching or abdominal pain to severe asthma or anaphylaxis. As milk becomes a less important part of the diet, the gut matures. Over time the allergic antibodies may disappear for good.

Conflicts About Food

Food is a serious preoccupation in modern society, both as a source of pleasure and as a source of anxiety. When you consider the epidemic of obesity that began in the United States and has now spread to other places that have adopted American-style diets, the confusion about the role of fat in diet, high carbs, low carbs, worries about refined foods, fertilizers, and food additives—the list goes on and on—it is understandable that something as misunderstood as allergy should take its place in the general mythology.

Worries about what is in our food go back a long way. When your authors were much younger and the addition of fluoride to water in order to combat tooth decay was commencing on a wide scale, some people thought it was a Communist plot.

In the 1960s we heard the expression "You are what you eat." Aggression and bellicosity—big preoccupations during the Vietnam War—were ascribed to consumption of processed foods and red meat. If only our leaders would become vegetarians, the logic went, it would put an end to war, which was amusing in light of the fact that Hitler was a vegetarian.

Today, with justifiable concern about an epidemic of eating disorders, we have fertile ground for another bout of hysteria, with food allergy as the enemy, which is a terrible shame because these allergies are real enough without embellishment. Phony food allergy wastes patient and doctor time, not to mention health care dollars. People with food phobias are easy marks for quacks. If they had real food allergies, however, they'd find their way to MDs soon enough, although not always the right MDs.

Hypochondria has always been with us, and allergy is rich territory for imagined ailments because it is so mysterious to most people. There are also quack psychiatrists who are anxious to attribute depression in people of all ages to food allergy. Parents who have trouble believing that their children's problems have true psychological or physiological roots sometimes like to believe that it's the food they eat.

"WE ANSWER TO A HIGHER AUTHORITY"

Hot dog eaters of a certain age will remember that as the tag line from an inspired commercial for Hebrew National. The point was that the rabbis who blessed their product had stricter standards than the FDA.

I thought about this not long ago when a small Orthodox boy suffered an anaphylactic reaction to a can of tuna. I questioned his family closely and had them bring in the can. Sure enough, it said *parve*, which means it is neither meat nor dairy, and it has not come in contact with either during preparation. This is something the parents, and indeed the markets that cater to their community, look for. Yet, it said clearly on the can that it contained casein as a preservative. Although I do not keep kosher except on the holidays, I have always respected the integrity of the rules as promulgated and enforced as immutable. For something containing casein to be labeled *parve* was a bit like finding out there were only nine commandments.

So I consulted a higher authority, the family rabbi. He informed me that *parve* only meant there was less than one-sixtieth by weight of milk. Well, that may be little enough for the rabbis, but it's still too much for a true food allergy.   — *Dr. Ehrlich*

FOOD ALLERGY: PERCEPTION AND REALITY

During my experience running a food allergy center, we encountered patients with food allergy complaints who did not have provable food reactions. They attributed vague and variable symptoms that occurred hours or even days after ingesting multiple foods to allergies, whereas real food allergies are manifest very shortly after eating a single food. The urge to blame life's problems on diet is powerful, and challenging it with medical science is really a challenge to a belief system. This is a great dilemma for the honest clinician. If the patient and the family are not adequately supported by, say a dietician and family therapist as well as an allergist while the food investigation proceeds, they may find their way to the nearest alternative practitioner, where food reactions that do not really exist will be treated with methods that do not work.   —*Dr. Chiaramonte*

Coming to Grips with Food Allergy

Interestingly, however, the fact that a child is severely allergic to one food doesn't mean he will be allergic to others. And while it's imperative that the child and his family be vigilant, even obsessive, about keeping the offending food away from him, it's also important to know what he is *not* allergic to.

Our children eat three times a day, minimum. They live active lives, we hope. They go lots of places and do lots of things, we hope. A severe food allergy casts a shadow across these activities. What should be a time of adventure and exploration becomes tentative. The limits we place on our children for their true allergies are bad enough. We shouldn't exaggerate them by casting too wide a net. This is another area where the insurance system can be penny-wise and pound-foolish whereas a certified allergist can be of tremendous help.

What Testing Doesn't Tell Us About Food Allergy

A *skin test* (in which a small amount of a suspected allergen is injected under the skin) or *RAST* (which involves blood analysis) with positive results in response to a food does not mean a person is allergic to the food. Allergy has to be confirmed by a challenge test. The patient may have the antibodies, yet be tolerant. A positive result may prompt a GP or pediatrician to recommend that those foods be avoided in addition to the peanuts, say, or milk, where the sensitivity is dangerous enough.

However, this technical sensitivity may not represent a problem that has to be handled with the same red-alert, DefCon-One vigilance as the primary concern. To stop with that test and rule out exposure to the whole range of foods categorically will have some pretty severe repercussions—financially, psychologically, experientially and even medically for the patient and the rest of her family.

Extending the same kind of protection necessary for the big allergies to these marginal sensitivities will make your child miserable. We don't want our food-allergic or asthmatic children for that matter to live in a bubble. A kid who can't enjoy the universal rite of passage of the peanut butter and jelly lunch shouldn't be deprived of the tuna sandwich with mayo just because a RAST shows sensitivity to fish or egg, which is in the mayo. Conversely, a kid who can't eat ice cream shouldn't go without peanut butter if he doesn't have to.

Much more beneficial to the patient, family, and extended family would be to see whether the child is allergic in the practical sense, or merely test-positive.

The gold standard is the placebo-controlled, double-blind challenge test (see chapter 7), which can be conducted only in an accredited food center. It is a long, cumbersome process, which can only be done one food per day.

These tests can be frightening to patients. They certainly don't want to experience the fear-of-death panic they associate with anaphylactic shock they may have experienced. Their parents don't want to witness it.

An experienced allergist can offer a middle way by applying a sample of the food to the skin, taking before and after pictures. If the first application doesn't react, we repeat the process on the lips without letting the patient ingest it. The final stage is full ingestion, with the doctor at the ready with epinephrine. By the time we get to this stage, we are pretty sure there will be no harm.

Even skillful doctors are reluctant to try this because insurance companies won't pay for it. This is very sad, because a negative challenge can save a person from a lifetime of difficulty. Running scared is ultimately much more expensive.

When dietary restrictions become burdensome, parents should insist on some sort of supervised food challenge. And if their insurance does not cover the challenge test, they should pay for it themselves. Measured by peace of mind and the possibility that they can stop working so hard to live within the strictures of the allergies, this will pay for itself many times over.

If the skin tests show positive reactions to kumquats most of the time, for example, the parents and the child can just avoid kumquats with no more study. How often does one eat kumquats anyway?

A frequently eaten food like wheat is another story. Avoiding wheat will alter the lifestyle of the child and family. Any food allergy that demands such drastic measures should be subject to a challenge test.

The odds favor some relief. Only about one-third of the skin-test-positive foods will be proven to cause allergic reactions on challenge tests. Challenge tests will show that some foods may be safely eaten in spite of the scratch test results.

Reading the Label Doesn't Always Help

You would think that with a long legacy of government regulation and the amount of money food manufacturers put into chemistry that they could come up with a reliable format for presenting accurate information on packaging.

Not so.

Misreading a label can be disastrous. In Dr. Sampson's study, all six deaths occurred because either the child or the parent was unaware the food contained a substance to which the child was allergic.

Parents of Food-Allergic Children conducted a study with parents visiting the pediatric allergy practice at the Mount Sinai School of Medicine. Parents were tested on how well they understood the ingredients listed on food labels. Only four of sixty parents of children with milk allergy, or 7 percent, were able to correctly identify the offending substances on fourteen products listing milk protein.

Anyone following a milk-free diet must avoid:

Artificial butter flavor
Butter, butter fat, buttermilk
Caseinates (ammonium,
    calcium, magnesium,
    potassium,
    sodium)
Cheese, cottage cheese, curds
Cream
Custard, pudding
Ghee (clarified butter used
    in Indian cooking)
Half-and-half

Hydrolysates (casein, milk
    protein, protein, whey,
    whey protein)
Lactalbumin, lactalbumin phosphate
Lactoglobulin
Milk (derivative, protein, solids,
    malted, condensed, evaporated,
    dry, whole, low-fat, nonfat, skim)
Sour cream, sour cream solids
Whey (delactosed, demineralized,
    protein concentrate)
Yogurt

Six of twenty-seven, or 22 percent, of parents of children with soy-restricted diets were able to correctly identify soy protein among nine products.

Anyone following a soy-free diet must avoid:

Akara

Hydrolyzed soy protein

Miso

Soy sauce

Soy grit

Soy nuts

Soy sprouts

Soy protein concentrates

Soy protein isolate

Tamari

Tempeh

Textured vegetable
protein

Tofu

Vegetable oil

Labels for wheat, egg, and peanut allergy–avoidance diets were also tested.

Anyone following a wheat-free diet must avoid:

Bread crumbs

Bran

Cereal

Couscous

Cracker meal

Enriched flour

Farina

Gluten

Graham flour

High-gluten flour

High-protein flour

Spelt

Vital gluten

Wheat bran

Wheat germ

Wheat gluten

Wheat malt

Wheat starch

Whole wheat flour

While most parents were able to correctly identify wheat or egg words on the ingredient labels, peanut was correctly identified by only forty-four of the eighty-two, or 54 percent, which is potentially disastrous considering the severity and longevity of peanut allergy. The most common error was parents missing the label statement "trace peanuts."

Anyone following a peanut-free diet must avoid:

Beer nuts	Peanut butter
Ground nuts	Peanut flour
Hydrolyzed vegetable protein	Peanut oil (cold-pressed,
Mixed nuts	expressed, or expelled)

If this is just beginning to give you an idea of how complicated a food allergy diet can be, look at the names that egg-allergics have to be able to spot.

Anyone on an egg-free diet must avoid foods that contain any of these ingredients:

Albumin	Livetin
Egg white	Lysozyme (used in Europe)
Egg yolk	Mayonnaise
Dried egg	Meringue
Egg powder	Ovalbumin
Egg solids	Ovomucin
Egg substitutes	Ovomucoid
Eggnog	Ovovitellin
Globulin	Simplesse

Anyone following a tree nut–free diet must avoid:

Almonds	Marzipan (almond paste)
Brazil nuts	Nougat
Cashews	Nu-Nuts (artificial nuts)
Chestnuts	Nut butters (cashew, almond)
Gianduja (a creamy mixture	Nut oil
of chopped toasted nuts in	Nut paste
high-quality chocolate)	Pecans
Hickory nuts	Pine nuts (pignoli, piñones)
Hazelnuts, including filberts	Pistachios
Macadamia nuts	Walnuts

This information on the interpretation of food labels by Parents of Food-Allergic Children is from the Food Allergy Initiative and the Food Allergy & Anaphylaxis Network. The FoodAllergy Initiative website is www.foodallergyinitiative.org. The Food Allergy & Anaphylaxis Network website is www.foodallergy.org.

Kicking the Prepared-Food Habit

A modern rule of thumb is that the healthiest family diet comes from shopping only around the periphery of the supermarket, where you find fresh produce, meat, and dairy. The internal aisles are where the processed foods lurk, with their ambiguous labels and hidden ingredients. This is a good rule for families with food allergies to follow.

One silver lining in the cloud of food allergy is that it may actually encourage families to rely more heavily on fresh ingredients and home cooking. After all, if you can't trust the labels, you have to go back to basics to control your child's diet. It may be time-consuming but it's a safer bet than relying on canned goods, junk food, or takeout. Besides, cooking can be fun. Cooking together and eating together are good ways to further cement the cooperative spirit of food allergy families. Even the youngest children can do their part safely, like mixing ingredients and tossing salads. Older kids can chop and cook.

Labeling Help

Time was when individual allergens had to be listed, but when a food was "standardized"—made according to an established formula—only the standardized food had to be listed. Thus, mayonnaise, which is made primarily of eggs and oil, was listed as mayonnaise, with extras like lemon juice listed separately. Not much help for an egg-allergic child who hasn't taken cooking lessons.

The late Senator Ted Kennedy of Massachusetts and Representative Nita Lowey of New York cosponsored the Food Allergen Consumer Protection Act several years ago. Senator Kennedy became interested in the field of allergy because one of the new generation of Kennedy children suffers from food allergies.

It is a pity that it takes some personal involvement for government to "get it," but that's the history of legislation.

Among the bills provisions:

• Products must list in common language any of the eight main food allergens: peanuts, tree nuts, fish, shellfish, eggs, milk, soy, and wheat. No chemistry set names like casein for milk components.

• An additive loophole was closed by requiring ingredient statements to take into account if any allergens were used in the spices, natural or artificial flavorings, additives, and colorings that are listed.

• Food manufacturers are required to include a working telephone number for information on food labeling.

• Food manufacturers are also required to better prevent cross-contamination between products produced in the same facility or on the same production line.

• The Centers for Disease Control and Prevention, a federal agency, is mandated to track the incidence of food anaphylaxis and death.

Postscript: Just as a matter of consumer prejudice, we never could figure out why manufacturers would use some of those technical words instead of the real names: Does casein really sound more appetizing than milk? Becoming a savvy reader of food labels is like learning another language. Food writer Michael Pollan has a simple rule of thumb for reading labels: Don't buy anything with more than five ingredients, or anything you can't pronounce. FAAN is working to create plain language requirements that could be adopted by the government. A substance like casein might become "casein (like milk)."

Will the issue ever be resolved? We agree: Not in our lifetimes. As long as food chemistry is regulated like food and not like chemistry, the industry will stay several steps ahead of consumer health.

Fresh Food Warning

Unfortunately, even fresh food can pose hazards. Casein is apparently used on produce and fish to maintain a fresh appearance.

Dining Out

There's nothing that a dedicated mother of an allergic child needs more than a good night out with the family and letting someone else do the cooking. Fat chance. For the family of an allergic child, it's like taking a Sunday stroll through a minefield.

Steve Taylor, PhD, head of the Department of Food Science and Technology at the University of Nebraska in Lincoln, says that restaurants are the biggest problem for people with food allergies.

Historically, restaurants have been regulated by local health departments and have not had to label foods. The problem is not the same as for mass producers of canned and packaged foods. "For many restaurants, labeling of food products they serve would cause horrendous problems," says Taylor. "What about chalkboard menus? How would you include all the ingredients? Enforcement would be a nightmare."

ON THE WOKS

Parents of a patient of mine who was peanut allergic had established an understanding with a neighborhood Chinese restaurant about their child, and usually had no trouble. But one night the boy took a bite of some Chinese food and threw up. Throwing up is good, parents: It means that the body is trying to expel the offending food. The chef heard about this and came out to discuss it with the parents. He finally realized that because a wok can be used to prepare one meal after another without intermediate cleaning, he decided to take special precautions. The next time the family came in, he showed them a special small wok that he would keep on the wall in the dining room and only use it for children with peanut allergies. The sight of that wok made the restaurant a magnet for families with peanut-allergic kids.

— Dr. Ehrlich

There's no easy way out of this. Restaurants are the archetypal small business. Maybe chains like McDonald's, which manufacture their food on the same industrial scale as Heinz or Dole, could be persuaded to avoid allergens—they are now listing calorie counts and avoiding transfats—but we wouldn't want to endorse the idea that making junk food safe for food-allergic children is any great boon to their health.

Individual action is exhausting. We have heard our parent support groups recount epic tales of the lengths they have gone to make a restaurant meal safe for their children. If you look at the list of egg-derived products above and anticipate going through it with a chef, even one who speaks English as a first language let alone the dozens of languages you hear in kitchens in large cities, and then repeating the process for milk, or legumes, or nuts, you can bet that maybe they're not going to make any money from feeding you no matter how many cocktails and bottles of wine you order—and at the end of this process, you're going to need them.

The problem is very real. At the FAAN 2001 conference, attendees were given a survey asking about their experiences in restaurants. The survey revealed a number of points:

• Almost half of these individuals have had an allergic reaction to a food served in a restaurant.

• The most common foods that caused the reactions were milk, peanuts, tree nuts, and eggs.

• Approximately 80 percent of participants avoid bakeries and Chinese and Thai restaurants.

• More than 70 percent of those responding reported avoiding ice cream establishments and Japanese and Indian restaurants.

• The most common concerns were: cross-contamination, lack of awareness by restaurant staff, and restaurant staff not taking food allergy seriously.

The best solution is education, and in this area, progress is being made. The Food Allergy Initiative (FAI) has given courses to restaurateurs for the kitchen and the dining area. We need to reward the restaurants that commit staff time to take these courses. Restaurateurs have a stake in this: Sooner or later the heavy hand of the tort bar is going to find its way into this, and lawsuits, well founded or not, will commence. In New York, famous old restaurants have gone out of business after a health code violation—think what would happen to a restaurant that sent a child to the hospital.

Other steps are being taken to better educate restaurant employees. The Food Allergy & Anaphylaxis Network and the American Academy of Allergy, Asthma and Immunology, along with the National Restaurant Association, produced a pamphlet on food allergies, which has been distributed to tens of thousands of association members. The brochure explains what restaurants can do to help customers who need to avoid certain foods, defines anaphylaxis, and advises employees what to do if food allergy incidents occur.

FOOD ALLERGY WATCH

Our friends and colleagues at the Food Allergy & Anaphylaxis Network are the great watchdogs on this subject. One of the most important features on its website, www.foodallergy.org, is "Special Allergy Alerts" (go directly to www.foodallergy.org/section/archives), which provides regular warnings on processed foods that have been recalled because of faulty labeling. Some sample alerts:

MILK AND PEANUT ALLERGY ALERT: August 31, 2009
Petri Baking Products Inc. is recalling "Stop & Shop Home Town Bakery Old Fashioned Molasses Cookies" due to undeclared milk and peanut.

The product was distributed to Stop & Shop stores in Connecticut, Maine, Massachusetts, New Hampshire, New Jersey, New York, and Rhode Island. The 8.9-oz. package bears UPC 6-88267-08457-7 and "sell by" date of Feb. 22, 2010 A. Consumers may return the product to the place of purchase for a full refund. Consumers with questions may call (800) 346-1981.

MILK ALLERGY ALERT: August 31, 2009
Chef Pierre ® is recalling "Chef Pierre Gourmet Lemon Meringue Pie" due to undeclared milk.

The product was distributed nationally. The package bears UPC 3210009293 and code 9159. Consumers may return the product to the place of purchase for a full refund. Consumers with questions may call (888) 891-6100.

EGG AND WHEAT ALLERGY ALERT: August 18, 2009
Shun Fung International Inc. dba, Yummy Foods Co., is recalling "Wife Cake" due to undeclared egg and wheat.

The product was distributed in California and Washington. The 17-oz. package bears UPC 0 19151 00168 2. Consumers may return the product to the place of purchase. Consumers with questions may call (415) 822-1768.

The "Special Allergy Alerts" section includes almost every cuisine we know.

At present the only treatment for food allergy besides the emergency injection of epinephrine is to avoid eating the food. Easier said than done. The Nutrition Labeling and Education Act has helped. So has training for restaurant staff. The FAI has supported research to develop simple test strips to check foods for common allergens.

Immunotherapy for Food Allergy?

How about altering the immune status of the food-allergic person? This was tried in peanut-allergic patients some years ago at National Jewish Hospital in Denver because peanuts are so difficult to avoid. A double-blind study of allergy shots with increasing amounts of peanuts with a salt-water control was attempted in two groups of peanut-allergic patients. Unfortunately, a patient who was in the salt water group received an injection of a strong peanut extract by mistake and died. The experiment was halted. The patients treated with the peanut extract were more resistant to allergic reactions from peanuts—not completely tolerant but less allergic. Without the mistake, the study might have been successful. Its revival is now under consideration.

Today, a number of approaches to immunotherapy are being studied, including anti-IgE injections, sublingual immunotherapy, and low-dose immunotherapy (see chapter 9, "Immunotherapy"). However, all these are in early stages of testing, and nowhere near adoption.

Genetic Engineering— Scientific Miracle or Frankenstein's Monster?

Genetic engineering of foods receives a great deal of publicity for the changes it might bring to the environment and the effects it might have on human health. Allergists view it as a double-edged sword. On the one hand, it may be possible to remove the allergens from food. On the other, allergens may be introduced into foods that are not currently allergenic. For example, some people who are allergic to tree nuts but not to soybeans might be adversely affected when genes from Brazil nuts are spliced into soybeans to enhance the nutritional value of the soy products, as has been done experimentally. Fortunately, this product never got to market for fear of what would happen to people who were allergic to Brazil nuts and ate the product. But this technology is still in its infancy.

There Must Be a Pony

A child's innate optimism is defined by the story about the little girl who comes down on Christmas morning, finds a pile of manure under the tree and starts squealing with joy.

Her mother says, "Why are you so excited?" The child answers, "With all this manure, there must be a pony somewhere around here."

In coming to grips with our children's allergies, we must try very hard to help them develop the internal resources to look on the bright side of their condition.

The Food Allergy & Anaphylaxis Network publishes a child's companion to its *Food Allergy News* called *Food Allergy News for Kids*, and one for teens as well, *Food Allergy News for Teens*. Both demonstrate just how resilient kids can be in the face of their condition.

A 7-year-old with a milk allergy says that by sitting at a special milk-free table in the school cafeteria at lunch, he manages to be the first one out the door for recess. A tree nut–allergic 9-year-old says she doesn't have to rush to get dessert at her school because her mother supplies a special one in a refrigerator in the cafeteria kitchen.

Indeed, by learning to take responsibility for their condition at an early age, children can acquire extraordinary problem-solving skills that can only serve them well as they get older.

One 12-year-old was fearful that she wouldn't be able to buy any snacks on a trip to an amusement park with her class, so she called the park and explained her plight. They sent a seventeen-page list of all the ingredients in every food sold at the park. Armed with this information, she could buy after all.

These newsletters publish not only the children's and teens' stories but their pictures as well. This is the basis of a peer community for youngsters who would otherwise feel isolated—they are truly not alone.

CHAPTER 6

Skin Allergies: Eczema, Hives, And Contact Dermatitis

Eczema—The Itch That Rashes

SOMETIMES WE WEAR OUR ALLERGIES ON OUR FACES—AND ARMS and legs. We are referring, of course, to eczema, which is also called *atopic dermatitis* (AD). It affects 8–15 percent of all infants and children, especially those with a strong family history of allergy, the majority of whom develop symptoms in the first year of life. The symptoms can be misleading: Those rosy cheeks that so many grandmothers want to pinch and which are traditionally considered healthy can be an early warning sign for eczema.

Eczema first appears as a rash and then as scaly, flaking dryness, and thickened skin that we describe as lichenification—a term that comes evokes lichens, the flaky vegetation you often see on rocks in the countryside. The course the disease takes with individuals is quite variable—mild cases go into remission by the age of 2 or 3, but more severe cases can persist on and off well into adulthood.

This inflammatory skin disorder may seem skin deep, but the misery it causes is not. What makes this disease so difficult for many children is how it affects the way they learn to relate to their own bodies, first physically, then psychologically. The itching cries out for scratching, and the scratching causes skin distress. That's why we refer to it as "the itch that rashes."

The preoccupation affects the way children deal with the world around them and how the world deals with them. Adults may notice the incessant scratching and probably admonish the child—futilely— to keep their hands off the rash. Over time, these children become objects of pity to grown-ups, and their parents become objects of scorn because they "don't do anything about it."

Other children can be fairly brutal about it. They notice first the scratching and then the accompanying disfigurement, and they may tease them about both. As eczema patients get older, the vanity component looms large in the way they see themselves. This vanity has repercussions well into adulthood.

THE DOCTOR'S WIFE

Sometimes I think the main reason my wife married an allergist was because of her own lifelong allergy problems, which, thanks be to God, and to good medical care, are now under control. I think of her as an attractive woman with four brothers and three sisters. One day I was looking at childhood pictures of her family. "Honey, I see your sisters. Where are your pictures? Do you have any baby pictures? Preferably naked."

"You dirty old man," she said, then added, "There are ... no pictures of me as a baby because my eczema was so bad that my parents hardly took any."
— *Dr. Chiaramonte*

Children with bad eczema sometimes find themselves relegated to the back row of family photographic portraits standing on chairs with the grownups when, by virtue of their age and height, they should be in the front. All these factors mean that eczema is not a superficial problem, but one that penetrates to the core of who they are.

Eczema often begins in infancy with dry patches, or a rash on the cheeks, face, and lower arms. As children get older, it affects the hands and areas where there are creases such as the *anticubital fossae* (in front of the elbows) and the *popliteal fossae* (behind the knees), and at the wrists.

The intense itching and scratching, often worse in the evening and during the night, keep the skin chafed and sometimes even weeping, oozing, and infected. Often the child with eczema leaves blood-stained sheets by morning because of all the scratching. Continual scratching can lead to the condition lichenification, which we described above. Scratching often enough and hard enough can lead to infected skin. The damage can become permanent. Both children and adults go to incredible lengths to achieve short-term relief. One adult we know will run his eczema-afflicted fingers under scalding hot water because it provides momentary relief, which he describes as "deep scratching." In fact, this is one of the worst things he can do because it dehydrates the skin so thoroughly that the itching returns with a vengeance.

However, if we can relieve the itching so that scratching is kept to a minimum, even the worst rash can often be made to disappear completely. If you control the itch, you can control the rash. Approximately one-half of all children with AD will lose their eczema before adulthood, and a majority of the rest have a good chance of controlling their symptoms.

> When I was a resident at Bellevue we used to tie children down and give them antihistamines to prevent them from scratching and keep the itch at bay. Many of them improved dramatically! That kind of treatment is no longer tolerated. We have to accomplish the same thing with medication. — *Dr. Ehrlich*

As with other kinds of allergies, eczema has its triggers, although it is usually difficult to determine the specific cause. Diagnosis is made on the basis of a physical examination and a thorough history. Unfortunately, laboratory tests are little help. However, the patient may have very high IgE (allergic antibody) levels. Most eczema patients have highly irritable skin so skin testing may not be advisable. Occasionally a RAST test may help pinpoint specific causes, but often, avoiding the specific cause does not become the whole answer.

The role of some airborne allergens in eczema is unclear, but there seems to be good evidence for that of dust mites and possibly other household allergens. Symptoms can be aggravated by heat and stress. Exposure to animals, animal-derived fabrics such as wool, and feathers can set off the itching.

In sensitive individuals, foods may have an effect, even if there is no other diagnosed food allergy. As with other food allergies, eggs, milk, peanuts, soy, wheat, or fish are the likely culprits with eczema, but other foods may also be at fault. If food is suspected, the physician may supervise removing the suspected foods from the diet for a trial period.

Skin care is an essential component to treatment. Moisture reduces itching. Soaking baths of cool water for twenty to thirty minutes twice daily are recommended, depending on the severity of the eczema. Soaking allows water to penetrate the outer layer of skin and actually "hydrate" it—making it moister. Just running water over it won't do. Bath oils must be used following the bath to retain moisture. When

Asthma Allergies Children: A Parent's Guide

RASH MOVE

Lindsay had red, rosy cheeks after she was born. What a cutie. At the age of 6 months she developed a red scaly rash on her face and later on the outer arms and legs. Lindsay frequently woke up at night crying and scratching. She was being bathed daily with Ivory Soap, which has the image of purity. Her parents tried baby lotion on the rash but this appeared to make rash worse. Then they tried Vaseline. And then after several difficult months, they tried a new pediatrician.

The doctor took a competent history. Significantly, Lindsay was breast-fed for three months, then was given Similac with iron, and when she developed colic, she was switched to Isomil. She was started on baby foods at 6 months of age and ate all types of baby foods along with some soft table foods such as mashed potatoes and carrots.

The new doctor asked if any foods seemed to make the rash worse.

"Maybe eggs," her mother replied, and then said, "but the skin is always so bad I could be wrong." Her father added, "Lindsay is so fussy now that it's hard to get her to eat anything."

The pediatrician placed Lindsay on a strict egg-free and milk-free diet. He recommended a moderate-strength steroid ointment for the dry itchy areas on the body and a milder cream for the facial areas. He also advised them how to remove allergens from the home. Lindsay improved considerably, and her problems were soon forgotten. Then at the age of 4, she developed a severe facial rash. It got so bad that kids at nursery school teased her and she no longer wanted to go.

Lindsay's parents were a modern egalitarian couple. The mother worked as a chief financial officer for a privately held company that held patents on a new line of pet pharmaceuticals. She kept cats and dogs at home to impress investors. The father, a professional contractor, stayed at home much of the time to look after Lindsay and her brother while running his business, and had recently undertaken an architecturally significant renovation of their home. This is not only when Lindsay's skin rash returned, but also when her nasal and chest problems began.

The pediatrician referred Lindsay to an allergist, who controlled the rash with antibiotics and Protopic, (continued on next page) a nonsteroidal immunosuppressive cream. He then undertook a series of skin tests because he felt they might motivate these driven parents to alter their lifestyles to benefit Lindsay. She was positive to molds, dust mites, cats, and dogs. Lindsay and her bother were sent to her grandparents while the father rushed to finish the reconstruction of the home. The mother removed the pets from the home; although she kept her job, she entertained investors elsewhere. Lindsay's skin rash improved dramatically along with the nasal and chest problems.

the child gets out of the tub, pat the skin dry and apply a lubricating cream within three minutes to seal in the moisture.

For smaller areas such as the elbows or behind the knees, which are prone to lichenification making it hard for moisture and medicine to penetrate, some doctors recommend washing and liberal doses of topical steroids covered by Saran wrap and held in place with an Ace bandage. This prevents any moisture from escaping while allowing the medication to do its work.

Eczema, like many other diseases, has a way of escalating from an acute condition (that is, one whose symptoms are short-lived) into a chronic one as patients seek short-term relief from annoying symptoms. Since the major problem is that the skin loses water and becomes very itchy, the scratching that follows allows the infection to penetrate deeper. The skin becomes inflamed to fight the infection which provokes more itching, more scratching, and further damage to the skin, allowing more water to escape and on and on.

Lotions containing alcohol should not be used because the alcohol will dry the skin. Also steer away from lubricants that contain lanolin, which is derived from sheep and thus may be allergenic, and paraben, a preservative that may sensitize the skin. The CVS pharmacy brand of lubricating cream is a good value and works well. For children with more severe AD, topical steroid creams prescribed by your physician can provide relief from symptoms and should be applied to the skin that has a visible rash as often as three or four times a day.

It is important not to apply steroid creams to unaffected areas—it increases adverse effects—or to the face without specific instruction from your allergist. Usually, a milder corticosteroid is used on the face as the rash improves. Your physician will prescribe the appropriate form of topical steroid. Other medications that may be helpful include antihistamines, which make the skin less itchy and, sometimes, antibiotics to clear an infection. The rashes of eczema result not from the disease itself, but from staph germs that infect the skin from the child's nails.

Atopic dermatitis comes and goes, and that can make it difficult to treat. Recognizing the early signs and working with your physician to identify triggers are keys to controlling it, but do not underestimate the importance of aggressive skin care at home such as baths and creams.

Protopic cream is a nonsteroidal, topical immunosuppressant for use in moderate to severe eczema that comes in two age-determined strengths: 0.03% (for children 2–15 years) and 0.1% (over 15 years). A major side effect is some tingling or burning of the skin. It is absorbed into the deeper layers of the skin and used twice a day.

Elidel cream is a nonsteroidal, topical immunosuppressant for use in mild to moderate eczema that comes in one strength and is used twice a day. There is little in the way of side effects and no tingling or burning of the skin. It is not absorbed into the deeper layers of the skin.

Medication Update

Elidel and Protopic both briefly became controversial when the FDA required that they be sold with "Black Box" warnings about side effects. In our opinion, the studies were flawed, the warnings were over-blown, and the drugs remain useful. They are particularly good for parts of the body such as the face, the eyelids, and the folds of the armpit and groin, where steroidal medications shouldn't be used routinely because the skin there is already thin, and steroids tend to make it thinner. They are also more expensive than older, generic drugs.

Tips for Eczema Housekeeping:

• Avoid using soaps on the skin—especially affected areas. Use cleansers such as Cetaphil when possible. Dove Soap, which used to be a fairly allergy-friendly soap, came out with a "hypo-allergenic" version, but it contained, of all things, almond oil, which is a terrible thing for a child with allergies.

• When doing laundry, avoid using fabric softeners or strong detergents.

• Wash clothes a second time without detergents.

• Dress your child in cotton clothes and use cotton sheets on her bed.

• On very hot days, discourage your child from too much strenuous activity. Sweat, like warm water, will dehydrate the skin when it evaporates, causing a rash we sometime refer to as "prickly heat," particularly in the front of the elbows and on the skin of the throat.

• If your infant is already scratching himself, you can slip cotton socks over his hands to keep from scratching.

• Keep your baby's fingernails short.

For more information contact: National Eczema Association, 4460 Redwood Highway, Suite 16D, San Rafael, CA 94903-1953. Call 800-818-7546 or log onto www.nationaleczema.org.

Wetting Your Child's Pajamas

Wet PJs conjure up one of the petty indignities of young families. However, Dr. Anne-Marie Irani of the Medical College of Virginia believes that wet PJs can be a good thing for children whose eczema is so bad that they can't stop scratching long enough to get a good night's sleep. You may have tried putting cotton socks on his hands, as suggested above, but they have come off and the scratching persists.

The itching of eczema is in part a function of severe dehydration of the skin as the immune system works overtime to combat allergy and infection. The fluids in the skin have been otherwise engaged, depriving them of their normal functionality of keeping the tissue moist.

In this case, Dr. Irani's answer is a variation on one of the world's ancient technologies—mummification. The object is to get the skin rehydrated long enough to stop the itching and provide relief.

Start with a warm bath to hydrate the skin. Then coat the afflicted areas with a layer of Vaseline to trap the moisture already in the skin. Wrap the area with cotton gauze.

Now, wet a pair of PJs, wring them out with your hands—you want them wet enough to compensate for the dehydrating effects of any perspiration overnight but not so wet as to be uncomfortable or chilling—and dress the child in them. Finally, put on another pair of dry PJs. According to Dr. Irani, a single night like this can restore the child's skin dramatically.

Bleach in the Bathwater

As we said, all that itching leads to scratching, and all that scratching leads to infection, which leads to more itching, scratching, and inflammation, which leads to ... well, you get the point. Our colleagues in dermatology at NYU recommend a familiar disinfectant, used in a novel way: Clorox. Add half a cup to a cup of Clorox to a bathtub of water for toddlers and up—for infants in a bathinette, use just an ounce—bathe with the face out of the water for ten minutes and then rinse with clean water. Results can be dramatic.

BAD NEWS FOR CAT LOVERS

While on a weekend in rural New Jersey near where my wife grew up, I met a family that was at their collective wits' end. Their 5-year-old son had been scratching nonstop for two years, it seemed. I reviewed their medications for eczema—there was nothing there that I wouldn't do. I even consulted a colleague of mine, a dermatologist at New York University School of Medicine. Then we visited their home. There was a beloved family cat who thought nothing of crawling into the boy's lap. He scratched the cat with one hand and scratched his face with the other. The cat had to go. It did. And the boy's condition improved rapidly. His eczema had nothing to do with New Jersey.   *— Dr. Ehrlich*

Hives, Still Mysterious

My teacher at Johns Hopkins said, "I'd rather have a tiger come into my office than a patient with chronic hives."   *— Dr. Chiaramonte*

Hives, or *urticaria*, is a distressing disorder that affects an estimated 20 percent of the population at one time or another. It is characterized by itchy, red, blanching on the surface of the skin. Urticarial lesions come and go and do not persist in a given location for more than 24 hours. The most common form of hives is known as "wheal-

and-flare," which may be a single red blotch or a cluster of them, and is triggered by the presence of an allergen in the area followed by the release of histamine when mast cells degranulate.

Most cases of urticaria are acute, lasting from a few hours to less than six weeks. In most acute cases, the trigger is obvious—a person eats strawberries or shrimp, for example, then develops urticaria within a short time.

Chronic Hives—What Causes Them?

Y ou may recall the great radio comedians Bob Elliott and Ray Goulding, known as Bob and Ray. Elliott is probably best known now for being the father of the comic movie actor Chris Elliott, but they were giants in the field. Every afternoon for many years, they regaled audiences with a particular brand of deadpan sketch humor that included "interviews" with some of the oddest characters you could imagine, played of course by one or the other.

One day, a "guest" came by whose claim to fame was that he had more allergies than anyone in the world. As they were speaking, the guest suddenly asked, "Is there a Tennessee walking horse in the studio?"

"No."

"Well, are there beaverboard Venetian blinds anywhere?"

No, again.

The guest pronounced with conviction, "There must be either a Tennessee walking horse or beaverboard Venetian blinds because I only get this particular hive with one or the other."

Hives can be mysterious, although perhaps not as mysterious as that, particularly in the case of those that last for periods over six weeks, which are classified as chronic.

Because there are so many possible causes, chronic cases require determined detective work on the part of the patient and physician. In some cases, the cause is never identified, and the hives usually just disappear with medical treatment. However, bouts of urticaria have been traced to such triggers as drugs (including aspirin), certain foods and additives, cold, sun exposure, insect stings, alcohol, exercise, endocrine disorders, infections, and emotional stress. In some people, pressure caused by belts and constricting clothing causes eruption.

Infectious triggers include the common cold, strep throat, and mononucleosis.

Patients who suffer recurrent episodes of acute urticaria, who have chronic urticaria, or urticaria complicated by swelling, trouble breathing, and other potentially serious problems should be formally evaluated by a specialist. A visit to your regular family physician is the first step in order to evaluate for nonallergic causes. If allergy is suspected, you will probably have to keep a diary containing such information as (1) foods your child has eaten, (2) any unusual exposures, and (3) when the hives appear. Bring the diary with you to the allergist's office.

To unravel the urticaria puzzle, the allergist-immunologist will take a detailed history about the patient's life, looking for clues that will help pinpoint the cause of symptoms. Frequency and severity of symptoms, family medical history, medications, work and home environment, and miscellaneous matters—these will all be part of the allergist's inquiry. The allergist will want to review your child's diary for further clues. In some cases your child may need blood and urine tests, x-rays, or other procedures. Skin testing may provide useful information only in some cases. The allergist-immunologist will decide which tests to order based on the different types of urticaria and the suspected cause.

I do remember learning about urticaria as an allergy-immunology fellow at Walter Reed Army Hospital, the famous military hospital near the nation's capital. The confusion about the problem was compounded by the fact that we were told that 80 percent of the cases we would evaluate would never reveal a cause. At one point my professor said something to the doctors that I repeat often to patients. He said, "For those of you who are going into practice and will treat urticaria I would suggest having an office with two doors to the outside." As we looked at him quizzically he continued, "You'll need one door for your patient to enter and the other for you to sneak out." His point was that there are many cases that defy diagnosis, it often takes a while before the right treatment is determined, and your patients are rarely satisfied with your treatment.

—*Dr. Ehrlich*

Two Categories of Hives: Allergic and Nonallergic

Allergic urticaria is less common than nonallergic, although it is somewhat more common in children than in adults. It is caused by the immune system's overreaction to foods, drugs, infections, and various substances. Foods such as eggs, nuts and shellfish, and medications such as penicillin and sulfa are common causes of allergic immunologic urticaria. Recent studies also suggest that some cases of chronic urticaria are caused by autoimmune mechanisms, when patients develop immune reactions to components of their own skin.

Nonallergic urticaria are those types of urticaria where a clear-cut allergic basis cannot be proven. These take many forms:

Dermographism ("skin writing") is an urticaria-like wheel that develops when the skin is stroked with a firm object like a blunt pencil. This can accompany other forms of allergy, but often is an isolated problem that comes and goes.

Cold-induced urticaria appears after a person is exposed to low temperatures, for example, when an ice cube is placed against the skin or after a plunge into a cold swimming pool or the ocean, which can actually be fatal if the throat swells up. Cold-induced urticaria is best treated with Periactin, an otherwise seldom used antihistamine.

Cholinergic urticaria, which is associated with exercise, hot showers, and anxiety, is a form of hives related to release of certain chemicals from parts of the autonomic, or involuntary, nervous system, which controls such body functions as blood pressure and heart rate.

Pressure urticaria develops from the constant pressure of constricting clothing such as sock bands, bra straps, belts, or other tight clothing.

Solar urticaria occurs on parts of the body exposed to the sun, often within a few minutes after exposure. This may be a reaction to drugs, such as doxycycline, months after taking them.

Cases of nonallergic urticaria may be caused by reactions to aspirin and, possibly, certain food dyes, sulfites, and other food additives.

In cases where the trigger for the problem can't be found, particularly with chronic urticaria, the condition is called *idiopathic urticaria*.

Where certain types of urticaria are more painful than itchy and leave bruises on the skin after they go away, a biopsy of the skin may be necessary for the diagnosis of autoimmune reactions.

Your allergist first will prescribe medications, such as the second-generation, less-sedating antihistamines Zyrtec and Clarinex, which are FDA-approved for use in hives, to alleviate the discomfort. Xyzal, a third-generation refinement of Zyrtec, is also very effective.

Histamine stimulates the production of stomach acids, and allergists have found that blocking its production may be helpful in hives. Oddly enough, on its face, this action of antihistamines is unconnected to the allergy-related action of the drugs. A class of drugs called histamine receptor antagonists, or H2 blockers, works by blocking the histamine receptors on the acid producing cells in the stomach, stopping one of the mechanisms by which acid is secreted. The old anti-ulcer medication Tagamet or even small doses of the antidepressant doxepin have this effect on acid production, which can make them useful for hives. Doxepin also has an anti-allergic, antihistaminic action. A leukotriene blocker such as Singulair, although not approved by the FDA for the treatment of urticaria, may help.

The best treatment for urticaria is to avoid the substance that triggers it. If a specific food is strongly suspected, don't eat it. Read the labels and ask in restaurants.

People with solar urticaria should wear protective clothing and apply sunscreen lotions when outdoors.

Loose-fitting clothing will help relieve pressure urticaria.

Avoid harsh soaps and frequent bathing to reduce the problem of

---

FUTURE TREATMENT?

A case recently came to our attention of a chronic asthmatic who had the good fortune (financially as well as medically, because the stuff costs $1,000 a month) to use Xolair. It helped not only with his asthma, but with his cold-induced urticaria. We can only speculate that this anti-IgE drug is functioning in the skin as well as the lungs. It makes sense to us, because cold can induce asthma in twitchy lungs. We doubt that this off-label use of Xolair will be transformed into an on-label use any time soon, not at current prices. But this is a reminder that allergic disease can be present in multiple parts of the body. We may one day find out that it's not just "one airway, one disease," but "one body, one disease."

dry skin, which can cause itching and scratching that can aggravate urticaria. Vigorous toweling after a bath may precipitate hives.

Although success in identifying the cause of chronic urticaria varies from clinic to clinic according to patient populations, it usually is no higher than 20 percent of cases. The good news is that with medical control of symptoms the hives usually disappear in time.

Contact Dermatitis—The Allergic Touch

Contact dermatitis, or "allergic eczematous contact dermatitis," results when sensitized individuals touch certain allergens or sensitizers. Unlike the typical allergic reaction seen in asthma, hay fever, food allergies and, occasionally hives, contact dermatitis involves a different part of the immune system and is called a "delayed hypersensitivity reaction."

The skin reactions are usually marked by a "weeping," red, bumpy, and very itchy rash. It looks like the rash poison ivy—nothing odd about that because poison ivy itself is a cause of this very condition. The rash may occur in a pattern that suggests its cause. When it occurs on the top of the foot, for example, the cause is probably chemicals used to cure shoe leather.

Many generations of campers have asked ruefully, Why are some people immune to poison ivy? Because they're not allergic to it, and the same is true for other topical allergens. The causes of contact dermatitis are many and varied, and as we continue to add chemicals into our lives from nail polish to face creams to adhesives

---

FACE THE FACTS

The symptoms of contact dermatitis are easily recognizable to trained eyes. My father, known to generations of Long Island children as Dr. Lennie, once pulled a drowning man out of the surf in the 1960s. He rushed into the sea and pulled the man to shore. As the man regained his strength, he looked at my father's face and said, "I assume you're not using makeup, so I must advise you not to use that suntan lotion." It was Dr. Alex Fisher, author of the definitive text on contact dermatitis. He gave my *(continued on next page)*

---

father an autographed copy of his book. What Dr. Fisher had noticed was a bumpy rash on my father's face that my dad was scratching, and hiving.

It is simple to assume that this rash is due to a contactant, i.e., an allergen exposed by contact, but many times one needs to be a sleuth to discover which one. Dr. Fisher assumed correctly that Dr. Lennie was not using makeup, and so he concluded, correctly so, that his suntan lotion must be the problem. Sometimes it's not so simple.

When I first went into practice, a very lovely 27-year-old woman came into my office, dressed to the nines, with an absolutely horrible, crusty rash on her eyelids. I first asked her if she stopped using makeup and, being the typical New Yorker that she was, she said, "Of course, I stopped using *everything*. Don't you think I would have thought about that before shelling out for 'a big specialist' like you?" She was rubbing her eyes furiously, and I was quickly losing her confidence.

Then I thought of the book *Contact Dermatitis* by Fisher. I showed her into the examining room, asked her to put on a gown while I quickly read up on eyelid dermatitis in my father's autographed copy—which I have in my office to this day.

Eyelid dermatitis, page 230. There it was in big, bold letters: *Eyelid dermatitis often is produced by cosmetics that are not directly applied to the eyelids (e.g., nail enamel).*

I put the book down, opened the door to the examining room, and looked down at her beautifully manicured nails. Eureka! I gave her rash a scholarly look and asked her to remove her nail polish and use nothing for the next few days. She was incredulous, but agreed to do so, and a call from her to my office two days later told me that the rash had resolved. What she was doing up to that time was continuously rubbing the enamel onto her eyelids, thereby provoking her dermatitis. It was a vicious cycle, which was aggravated by the fact that she would try to make herself feel better by treating herself every week with a manicure and a professional polish job. Simple patch testing with these chemicals confirmed the diagnosis. Thank you, Alex.

—*Dr. Ehrlich*

and the like there will be those who may become sensitive to them.

Because of incidents like that, allergists should always inquire about various chemicals and how they "touched" the skin. Fisher's book is a trove of information about the effects of particular items in the formation of contact dermatitis. Nickel, for example—a common element in gold earrings, rings, and, of course, coins—produces nickel dermatitis. In fact, as reported in the Science section of the *New York Times* in September 2002, Swiss scientists were predicting a large increase in contact dermatitis because of the design of the new Euro-denominated coins in European monetary union countries as the coins begin to wear down from regular use. The Swiss do not use the Euro but as experts in both pharmaceuticals and money, they keep on top of both subjects.

Ammonia in diapers and chemicals in clothing are also prominent on the list. And, of course, there's poison ivy. It all seems so obvious if one asks the right questions and observes the location of the rash. You may have seen an episode of the television show *ER* in which Dr. Greene contracted a virulent rash on a very intimate part of his body. It turned out that his wife had touched him affectionately after berry picking in the woods during a camping trip.

On-the-spot testing for the exact causes of a particular case is complicated by the fact that it is unlikely an allergist will have all the likely substances that cause it in the office at any particular time. An international committee on this problem has come up with the true test: twenty-two mixtures of common contact allergens, plus controls, on two large adhesive strips placed on the back of the patient for 48 hours. The necessity to test is rare enough that we have to order these ahead of time.

Of course the first treatment for this rash is to stop contact with the allergen. The true test kit has advice on how to accomplish this but in some cases it is impossible to cease all contact, as in the case of handling coins. After all, nickel is added to all of them to harden softer metals.

The more difficult cases of contact dermatitis must be treated with corticosteroid cream, and the patient's parent should consult a specialist for patch testing. Most dermatologists and some allergists will surely be of help.

CHAPTER 7

Testing, Testing, 1-2-3 Testing: What is Your Child Allergic To?

ONE TOPIC IN MEDICINE THAT HAS HEATED UP SINCE WE FIRST published this book is the lost art of clinical diagnosis. Doctors in training have come to rely so heavily on technology that they fail to develop their powers of observing and listening to patients. *House*, the popular TV program, is built around the issue. Dr. Lisa Sanders of Yale (where Dr. Chiaramonte trained long ago), whose *New York Times Magazine* column "Diagnosis" inspired the show, has chronicled the erosion of diagnostic skills in part because doctors cannot see the forest for the tests. Another doctor says that the joke at his hospital is that the residents need a CT scan, blood tests, and an MRI before they will call a broken arm a broken arm.

In the field of allergy, we have been beating this drum for a long time. To the specialist's eye, much testing is beside the point, and can lead to wrong conclusions.

Wait a minute! Can't you find IgE in a test tube? What do you need an allergist for? Can't a GP read a printout from a blood sample as easily as a specialist?

Well, yes and no. Yes, a GP can read the lab reports showing, say, that a patient has allergic antibodies to pollen and nuts, but not to cat dander, or any number of other combinations. However, the bigger question is whether the tests conflict with or support the patient's history, or whether the expense and time involved could have been avoided just by listening to the patient with a trained ear. The science is there, but you don't have to look at all the molecules every time.

The science shows us that skin tests and blood tests don't really measure the same things. The antibodies that register in a blood test have a half-life of two days. They come and go without putting your immune system on a state of red alert. The ones that react in the skin have a half-life of six to eight weeks, which means that your body is ready to strike for a protracted period. Thus, you may control one sneezing fit with an antihistamine, but as soon as the medication wears off, you will start blasting away immediately.

False Positives and False Priorities

Patients are rarely allergic to more than three or four major foods, yet RAST tests will frequently register many more. Two-thirds of skin tests will also register positives that don't stand up under double-blind food challenges. Yet, anxious parents, armed with a positive blood or skin test, will frequently err on the side of caution and exclude all the offending food groups. The result is essentially malnutrition. Our practices regularly see two or three new patients per month who have "dropped off the growth curve." That is, they are not getting enough nutrition to keep up with their peers physically or, presumably, mentally.

PEARLMAN OF WISDOM

When I was training, I had a mentor named Alan Pearlman who told me,"I never test for allergies." I thought he was crazy. Well, if he was, then I am almost crazy, because I test less and less.

As you develop clinical experience, you find that a good history is much more important than any lab report. Sometimes I will test to confirm what I already suspect.

Patients and parents of patients don't always like this. They will say, "If you don't test, what am I paying you for?" I tell them, "You are paying me to use all my experience to make you (or your child) better."

— *Dr. Chiaramonte*

Given the economics of medicine, this situation is not likely to turn around quickly: Tests can be billed for. Dr. Sanders is very direct on the subject: "Doctors are paid to do, not to think."

Our insurance system is penny-wise and pound-foolish. A visit to an allergist is more expensive than one to a gatekeeper physician, but when you add up the serial costs of follow-ups to the gatekeeper, the payment to the allergist starts to look cheaper. When you throw in unnecessary tests and mistaken treatments, the costs are higher still. Legislators complain about unnecessary testing and the high cost of medical care. Allergy is a case in point—a lot of money gets spent that might not have to be. Add in the question of patient misery, which can't be measured. "Series of scratch tests—$1,000. Emergency hospitalization—$7,000. Childhood saved from perpetual coughing, wheezing, sneezing, and overall discomfort—priceless." A good allergist will test 10 percent of the time.

As we mention in chapter 1, the ranks of allergy specialists are thinning, and the economics of health care are squeezing more and more out of primary care physicians. That is why we are trying to disseminate more of what we do more widely, to help our colleagues in the overworked primary care specialties, as well as concerned parents.

Much as we want parents and patients to be "informed consumers," we don't want them to think that getting good value for their money requires laboratory results and computer printouts. They can be as meaningless as phrenology.

Research Bearing Fruit

The story is not all bleak by any means. While we personally regret that some allergists in training are headed for the laboratory instead of the examining room, there's no question that they are doing good work that will help doctors and patients. One exciting development is that specific allergens can be isolated in food, which leads to more specific testing, and eventually, we hope, more effective targeted therapies.

A Good History Solves the Mystery

Allergy tests are very important, but they are often not necessary. A very substantial proportion of the time, they could be avoided through a thorough history by a good allergist who knows what questions to ask, which ones not to ask, and how to interpret the information provided by the patient or the patient's parents.

This is the kind of history that gatekeeper physicians are just not equipped to discover, even if they have a detailed knowledge of allergy. They try to match symptoms with treatment as best they can, but usually do not establish cause and effect with the complex array of environmental and behavioral factors that can contribute to allergies. Their method is more likely to involve trial and error than probability. While science in the form of chemistry is still the most important answer much of the time, there are other things at work that contribute to allergic attack or stand in the way of effective use of needed drugs.

Depending on the age of the child—or the adult for that matter—testing patients is annoying, boring, and, when needles are involved, painful and scary. For those reasons, we try to minimize our reliance on certain tests. In any case, our first preference as allergists is always to rely on our own clinical experience and judgment, with testing as an adjunct.

For example, a test may show sensitivity to cats. Scientists have isolated a single protein as the culprit in cat allergy. That protein, dispersed throughout a cat owner's home in saliva, dander, and cat by-products, causes a variety of symptoms from itchy skin and burning eyes to rhinitis (stuffy nose) and asthma. These range, of course, from the merely annoying to the life threatening.

You don't have to be as cynical as TV's Dr. House, who thinks that patients *always* lie, to acknowledge that patients and their parents are not always the most reliable witnesses to their own lives, particularly when it comes to pets. When you ask some patients if they in fact have a cat in the home, they will lie about it, probably because they are afraid the doctor will tell them get rid of it.

We're all human, and sometimes people can't bring themselves to act on their good sense. Allergic cat lovers will put up with all kind of misery. Their mates are not always so tolerant, however. We have seen in clinical practice a nonallergic spouse, after all else fails, file for divorce rather than give up a cat. Children all over the country have been left heartbroken as their parents were forced to choose between their health and their pets. You can imagine then the huge interest among allergic cat lovers in genomic research, which might replace this gene with a nonallergic substitute, leading to the breeding of an allergy-safe cat.

We bring this up because it demonstrates how intertwined the human misery and suffering caused by allergies are with the frontiers of science on the one hand, and some very primitive emotions on the other. And certainly, science is a big part of the story throughout the field of allergy. As you will learn in chapter 8, treatment today is heavily dependent on chemistry.

However, the critical role played by laboratory science is frequently not as important as good old physician experience and solid clinical medicine when it comes to making a good diagnosis. An allergist who suspects "cat" will not take no for an answer, even without skin scratches and other tests.

Sherlock Holmes

"You have come by train this morning, I see."

"You know me, then?"

"No, but I observe the second half of a return ticket in the palm of your left glove. You must have started early, and yet you had a good drive in a dog-cart, along heavy roads, before you reached the station."

The lady gave a violent start and stared in bewilderment at my companion.

"There is no mystery, my dear madam," said he, smiling. "The left arm of your jacket is spattered with mud in no less than seven places. The marks are perfectly fresh. There is no vehicle save a dog-cart which throws up mud in that way, and then only when you sit on the left-hand side of the driver."

— *Sir Arthur Conan Doyle,*
The Adventure of the Speckled Band

Conan Doyle was a 26-year-old physician when he created Holmes, but Holmes's method was modeled on Doyle's medical school instructor Dr. Joseph Bell, who would astonish his students with his observational and analytical abilities.

You can see the medical process at work in every Sherlock Homes story. At the first meeting between Holmes and his client in each, you will read what could easily be an allergic medical history, except that the subject is murder, mayhem, or blackmail instead of itching, sneezing, or wheezing.

Holmes puts his overanxious clients at ease by letting them tell their stories, with the occasional interruption to ask a specific question on one point or another. While he may not have solved the mystery by the end of the interview, he would at least have framed the issues and directed the inquiry so that it can be solved, saving lives, fortunes, and peace of mind in the process, or—in medical terms—so that "treatment" can commence.

Sometimes we allergists do solve the mystery in that initial interview. But as with Holmes, by way of Yogi Berra, the story ain't over till it's over. We need to treat the patient.

The Right Questions Often Answer Themselves

When you go to your GP's office, you know enough to take something to read in the reception area. Then you usually go to an examining room for a time while you wait for the physician to finish a previous consultation. In this beehive environment, most overworked doctors have no time for what are called "nondirective questions," which elicit both perceptions about their lives as well as nuggets of information. For example: "What's going on in your life?" or "Why are you here?"

Most patients are pretty disciplined about keeping their answers pertinent to the issue of their health, which allows us to ask further questions such as:

"What makes it worse?" "What makes it better?" "What do you think about your problem?"

After the nondirective questions, we then can ask more directive questions, because we now know what the patient thinks.

Well, it doesn't take all day, but it does take a considerable amount of time. Usually the patient—or in the case of pediatric allergy, the patient's parent—has some ideas about whatever it is that's precipitating the current misery. Those ideas may be wrong. They might attribute their current difficulties to pollen instead of a pet, but in telling the full story, the real contributing factors tend to come out.

New schools, new homes, new activities, new pets, new foods, new beds, even new *boyfriends* or *girlfriends*—all these can be key clues to the onset of allergy, recurrence, or worsening allergic condition.

For example, someone might move into an older building and six months later their kids start to exhibit allergic symptoms. Is there evidence of mice or roaches?—a sensitive subject because it reflects on mom and dad's housekeeping habits. Any kind of vermin is likely to provoke allergy. Conversely, it might be a *brand new* house. We might ask whether there is any evidence of water damage. If the answer is yes, there might be mold, which means that the family shelled out a big pile of money for a house that leaks.

Sometimes allergies get worse after a family gets rid of the cat. Why? Because the cat caught the mice, and the mouse droppings are worse than the cat.

Sometimes the clues lie not in what people say but in their body language. If they're afraid the doctor will give them advice they don't want to hear, that little Rambo has to go, for example, something in their manner may come across as uncomfortable or evasive.

And yet, the information they withhold because they don't want to deal with bad news can be catastrophic.

Who Is the Culprit?

One of the most common problems we encounter when a GP refers a patient to us is that the culprit is the patient himself. The problem is frequently that he has gotten better temporarily and then regressed. Or in spite of regular treatment there are still periodic emergency room visits.

In cases like this, one of the most important things an allergist can do is find out what medications the patient is on, the schedule on which they are to be taken, and which ones seem to work. We frequently find that patients suffer from medication fatigue. They simply get tired of

---

TRAGIC DENIAL

I had a patient who was repeatedly hospitalized from the age of 2 weeks to the age of 2 months. I couldn't figure out why she kept having relapses. The mother repeatedly denied having any pets. She also said her house was in good shape. Finally, I took a nurse with me to make a house visit. Not only were there a St. Bernard and a cat in the house, but the ceilings were discolored from leakage around the windows. I told her she had to get rid of the pets and have the windows and siding replaced. The next day I got a call from her saying that a pulmonologist—lung specialist—she knew said he could cure the child with no major change in the home. Three weeks later the child was dead.   — *Dr. Chiaramonte*

---

taking it. An asthmatic may be on a regimen of an inhalable steroid with an inhaler as back up. But the daily inhalable steroid requires discipline for effective use, while the rescue inhaler provides instant relief. No wonder then that patients will slide on the use of the steroid—after all, regular use is a constant reminder that he has asthma—and then resort to the inhaler in an emergency. This provides temporary relief, but then it has to be used again—three or more times a day in many cases—and each time it provides instant relief.

What's wrong with that, you may ask, if both get the job done?

The answer is that while both work they are not equal treatments. The inhaler is a stronger drug, which provides a jolt to the system that over time will hurt you. Then too, there's the cumulative damage to the lungs from repeated inflammation. The steroid keeps this at bay by staving off the inflammation. Regardless, anything that sends you to an emergency room three or four times a year can't be good for you.

Shrinking from the Truth

Dr. House on television says, "Everyone lies." While we are not as cynical as he is, we are fully aware that patients aren't always as forthcoming as they should be. But why would anyone withhold valuable information from a doctor? This is really a question for a shrink—a psychotherapist. The reasons are as varied as the individual patients. Sometimes, as we have discussed, it's the love of a pet. Sometimes it's because they're afraid of the financial cost of change, which is certainly the case if the allergen is in the walls, ceilings, or foundation of the home. Sometimes it's because they have bad habits—smoking would be an example, although not, we would hope, for any of our pediatric patients—or because they don't clean their homes thoroughly. Their parents are, of course, another matter.

Sometimes it's because they are wary about the medication. As we have said, this is particularly the case with steroids because athletes have given steroids a bad name, even though they're not the same kind of drug.

Sometimes the answer is psychologically complex. The illness defines their existence—they might be afraid of getting better because they would then have the problem of finding out what to do if they were healthy.

Regardless of these or any other reasons, convincing them to change their habits, to take their medication and make any of the other lifestyle changes that are a part of an allergy-free life takes time, education, and discipline. For kids, it also takes a support system of parents, friends, and medical practitioners who can encourage them to hang in there.

When you read Sherlock Holmes, while you get the idea that he has solved most of the mystery in that initial interview, the story doesn't end there; if it did we would need to find something else to read. We still have the pleasure of reading as he solves the mystery.

The allergy story doesn't end with the history either, although unfortunately the rest of it is not as entertaining as Holmes. Sometimes the doctor's judgment has to be backed with courses of testing, if only to convince a skeptical patient that there is indeed a problem. Finding the right level and regimen of medications may indeed take some trial and error. To return momentarily to the subject of science, the science of allergy is good and getting better. But it will have to be a lot better before we can rely on science alone to treat allergy. In the meantime, we have to rely on good information, much of it anecdotal, and most of it from patients and their parents. That all starts with the history.

That's not to say that testing is irrelevant. Hardly. It is critical to understanding current levels of disease, particularly the home-administered monitoring that goes on with asthma. In other cases, such as food tolerance, tests are invaluable for reinforcing the importance of continued treatment, or ascertaining when treatment might end. Finally, they can be very helpful in determining which allergens to introduce during immunotherapy.

Still, not all doctors who employ these tests have a detailed understanding of the procedures or their strengths or weaknesses as diagnostic tools, not to mention the nuances of allergy itself. They will order the tests anyway, and administer them without detailed discussion with the patient's parents of what's involved or what they are looking for.

Allergy Tests

Skin Tests: These are the classic tests that spring to mind when the search for allergenic causes of asthma, hay fever, or eczema begins. The test involves pricking or scratching the skin and then applying possible allergy-provoking substances. If a patient is allergic, the allergen will look like a mosquito bite. Sometimes this may be followed up with an *intradermal* test below the skin. As we have said elsewhere in this volume, the tendency is to overtest, which is to order tests that are probably superfluous if a good medical history is taken. These also fall under the heading of annoying because they leave the patient with railroad-tracks of itching up and down their forearms. An alternative to the intradermal test is the *percutaneous* test or "prick" test which is much faster and less painful.

WEDDING BELL BLUES?

While children would rather not be "stuck" at all, this method of testing can be done with a minimum of pain and reveal a great deal of information very quickly. Reggie Jackson once said the typical New Yorker asks only one thing: "What have you done for me in the last ten minutes?" A mother once came to my office on a Friday morning bringing her daughter in as a new patient. They were attending a wedding the next day at a friend's weekend house where there were cats, and the patient was the maid-of-honor. We knew from her history that the child was allergic to dogs, but her mother wanted to know about cats because she did not want to risk her 12-year-old having an allergic reaction. She would skip the wedding instead. Oh yes, by the way, she could be tested, but was wearing a sleeveless dress, and there could be no marks on her arm.

Skin testing was performed on the inner thigh, she was negative, and the wedding went off without a hitch.   — *Dr. Ehrlich*

Radioallergosorbent (RAST) Tests: Instead of directly testing the skin, these involve drawing blood to detect the presence of IgE antibodies. The advantage is that multiple causes of allergy and asthma can be detected without repeated scratching, although RAST is not as accurate as direct skin testing. However, for young children it may be preferable to have a single blood letting than repeated skin tests. In cases of bad eczema, furthermore, the skin may not tolerate direct testing.

ImmunoCAP ISAC: This is the latest thing in testing. Developed by VBC Genomics and Phadia, ImmunoCAP uses specific molecular components of allergens. Conventional testing uses are based on aller-

---

COMMONSENSE TEST

RAST tests are easy to do. Too easy. Many primary care physicians pick the tests to be done like throwing darts or just check off everything.

In one instance, we reviewed the case of an Orthodox Jewish 9-year-old child whose doctor checked off every food from A to Y (apple to yam). The insurance company was paying for the tests and rightly demanded an explanation from the doctor. The reasoning was weak to begin with, but absolutely fell apart when an astute insurance adjuster—there are some—asked, "Why pork?"

A history taken by a trained allergist—even a non-Jewish one—would have eliminated many needless tests.

In other words, RAST testing may show us a forest when we want to see individual trees. ImmunoCAP can show us the trees.

We must point out, however, that diagnosis is only half the story. Treatment is another matter.   — *Drs. Chiaramonte and Ehrlich*

---

gen prepared from biological raw materials, which contain mixtures of allergenic and non-allergenic molecules. They can't be fully standardized according to major or minor allergen components, which may account for some of the false positives we see in RAST testing, as in the following case.

The number of components ImmunoCAP can test for now is limited but growing. The big test will come when we see if it leads to more precise therapies. However, one advantage to anxious parents and children is that it involved only a fingertip prick instead of blood drawing or skin scratching.

Patch Tests: These are done to determine whether contact with a particular substance is the cause of a skin condition, say a rash that may come from wearing certain earrings. An adhesive patch containing various potentially allergenic substances, such as preservatives and dyes, is placed on the skin, usually on the back. The patch is removed after 48 to 72 hours. A small skin rash similar to poison ivy will indicate contact allergy.

Oral Challenge: As also described in our chapter on food allergy, oral challenge is indicated where skin testing is not definitive about the extent of a problem with certain foods—or drugs for that matter. For example, a food may register positive in skin testing, but the patient can actually tolerate it because he has outgrown the problem, as often happens with milk. Because of the potential for anaphylaxis, it is done in an office or hospital where emergency medicines and equipment are on hand. Small amounts of a substance are given. The patient is monitored for symptoms such as wheezing, hives, or decreased blood pressure. The "gold standard" test is the double-blind, placebo-controlled food challenge. This test involves "blinding" both the patient and the investigator from seeing what the patient is getting so that there are no false reactions. The test is cumbersome and therefore reserved only for special facilities. It is very accurate. If there is no reaction, quantities are increased gradually until a normal dietary amount or full dose of the food or drug are given.

NUTS TO YOU

I once had a 14-year-old child return to my office for a follow-up visit to see if he still had an allergy to nuts, and specifically, pecans. While waiting to see me, an old family friend whom he hadn't seen for a long time walked in, and when they saw each other embraced and kissed.

My nurse called me into her examination room where the teenager was having an anaphylactic reaction. We were perplexed until the friend ran in from the waiting room and blurted out that she had had *pecan pie* for lunch. The young man was treated and watched for four hours in the office. The "test" was considered positive as an oral challenge. (No the insurance would not cover it!)

— *Dr. Ehrlich*

Tests of Immune System Function

In some cases, asthma, eczema, or other allergic conditions may be connected to abnormalities in the larger infection-fighting immune system. The symptoms may include allergies or asthma that are exceptionally severe, difficult to control, or that appear along with unusual or repeated infections.

Complete Blood Count (CBC): The most comprehensive test of the immune system, this measures white blood cells, platelets, which are involved in clotting, and hematocrit—the concentration of blood. The white blood cell count is often examined under a microscope to determine levels of these cells:

• Lymphocytes, such as T and B cells, direct the entire immune system and make antibodies to fight infections.

• Neutrophils, cells normally seen in pus, are the first line of attack against invading bacteria and other infections.

• Eosinophils, usually found in very small quantities, are known to be important in allergic disease such as asthma or drug allergies. They are also elevated with conditions such as systemic lupus, cancer, or parasitic infection.

• Basophils, similar to eosinophils, can also be found in allergic and other diseases.

Immunoglobulin (Antibody) Levels: These are proteins the immune system produces to fight infection, which we discussed in an earlier chapter. They come in four classes: Immunoglobulin (Ig) G, A, M, and E. The test usually involves taking a small amount of blood and comparing antibody levels to standard levels for age.

• IgG is the main antibody in fighting blood-borne infections. Low levels are seen in a condition known as common variable immunodeficiency, which often causes recurrent pneumonia, sinus disease, and difficult-to-treat asthma.

• IgA is the antibody involved in protecting the lining of the digestive, respiratory, and reproductive systems. Although this is the most common antibody deficiency (1 in 400 persons), deficiencies usually only cause mild symptoms including recurrent sinus infections.

• IgM is the first antibody that turns out to fight an infection. It is then replaced by longer-lived IgG . The immune system uses this antibody to activate the complement system, a sequences of interactions that bring about inflammation and other immune responses that help eliminate infections. A rare immune disease called hyper-IgM syndrome involves the inability to shift from IgM to the other antibody types. The blood shows extremely high levels of IgM and low levels of the other antibodies. The hallmark of low antibody levels is recurrent infection.

• IgE, as mentioned earlier, is the main antibody seen in allergic disease. Its primary role is thought to be defending against parasites. Levels are often checked to determine the degree of allergy or atopy a patient has. Elevated levels often correlate with severe eczema.

Specific Antibody Levels (Recall Titers): When people are success-fully immunized against an infectious agent, these tests should show a measurable presence of antibodies to specific organisms such as measles virus or tetanus. This is a *qualitative* test as it deter-mines how well the B cell or *humoral* system functions. (See *lymphocytes*, above.)

Delayed Hypersensitivity (TB or candida skin tests): After exposure to certain infections, the body may produce T cells that can respond the next time to stop subsequent invasions. This test is a descendant of the old tine test, and utilizes either the familiar PPD tuberculin, or candida, mumps, or other substances that most people have been exposed to at one time in their lives. The process involves injecting a few drops under the skin, usually on the forearm. The physician observes the site in 72 hours for a reaction. In a normally functioning immune system, the candida or mumps sites should show a raised, red area. This test is also qualitative as it determines the function of the T cell or *cell-mediated* system. (See *lymphocytes*.)

Lymphocyte Proliferation Assay (or Mitogen Assay): Another qualitative test of the immune system, this assay is usually done in highly specialized research labs. It involves removing a patient's white blood cells from a blood sample and exposing them to certain substances known as *mitogens*. If the cells are working normally, mitogen exposure will cause them to divide or proliferate to a degree that can be compared to a standard. In certain immune diseases there is a lack of ability to respond properly, thus leading to infections.

Testing for related conditions: As the adage says, "All that wheezes is not asthma," and conditions that are not strictly allergic or immunologic may play a role in symptoms similar to those of asthma. To this end, the physician may perform certain tests or refer the patient to a specialist for further evaluation. Some of the tests involved in determining other diagnoses that cause asthmatic symptoms are described next.

It should be noted that not all these tests are performed by the specialist. After a careful history and physical, they can be used by a primary care physician to confirm elements of a preliminary diagnosis.

Tests of Breathing

Peak Flow Measurement: This is one of the simplest and most useful tests, both in the office and often at home. The test involves blowing into a handheld device that gives a numerical reading called a peak flow rate, usually expressed in liters per minute. This helps determine how well asthma is controlled. If used daily, it can give an early warning of worsening asthma. As doctors, we love it because we can determine over the phone whether the child is truly having a problem with his or her asthma and subsequently monitor his or her progress without necessarily having to examine the child. Simple as they are, however, they must be obtained through a doctor and instruction must be given in their use.

Pulmonary Function Tests: Also known as *spirometry*, this test is usually done in the office of either an allergist or a pulmonologist. It is a more sophisticated evaluation of the lungs and is often used to make a definitive diagnosis of asthma. The test involves breathing into a machine that calculates different breathing parameters. By testing before and after giving the patient an inhaler such as albuterol, the clinician can see if there is significant improvement. Improvement may indicate reactive airways as found in asthma. The test is limited by its difficulty to perform in children less than 6 years old.

Exhaled Nitric Oxide (eNO) Test: As discussed in chapter 3, eNO is a marker for inflammation in the lungs. A patient may not have asthma symptoms but still have elevated levels of inflammation, which can damage the lungs unless controlled. After the patient exhales into a portable device, the doctor can get an instant reading on the degree of inflammation.

Imaging Tests

Chest X-Ray/Sinus X-Ray: Also known as radiographs or roentgenograms, these tests may be done in the office or at a hospital or radiology facility. These tests involve a small amount of radiation focused on a film, and take only a few minutes to perform. They will show tissue irregularities such as pneumonia in the lungs or sinus disease.

CT (CAT) Scan: This test utilizes computers to enhance radiographs and give much more detail. It involves lying on a table and being moved through a ring while images are made, a process that often can be done in less than fifteen minutes. This test is especially helpful in viewing sinuses and determining if they are chronically affected.

Sweat Test: In patients who have breathing problems associated with repeated pneumonia, poor growth, and problems with digestion, the condition known as cystic fibrosis (CF) must be ruled out. As this condition involves problems with salt in secretions, testing involves determining the salt concentration in sweat. Extremely high levels in a patient described as above are concerning for CF.

The pH Probe and Milk Scan: In some cases asthma symptoms may occur when food travels in the wrong direction from the stomach backwards into the food tube or *esophagus*. This is gastroesophageal reflux disease (GERD). Usually evaluated by a gastroenterologist, a specialist in disorders of digestion, this condition is tested in two ways. In older children and adults the pH probe test involves measuring stomach acid in the esophagus over a 24-hour period using a device that senses changes in the acidity or pH of the esophagus. In younger children where this test may not be feasible, a test known as a milk scan may be performed. Usually performed by a radiologist in a hospital or outpatient radiology center, the test involves having the child swallow a substance such as milk with markers so it can be traced. Images of the food tube are made over time and the radiologist can determine if there is reflux of the food into the mouth or airway. These tests can aid in treatment of GERD and associated breathing problems.

Echocardiogram: In some cases wheezing or other asthmatic symptoms may have a heart-related or *cardiac* component. If an underlying heart condition is suspected, the physician may recommend a test known as a cardiac ultrasound or echocardiogram. Usually performed by a heart specialist known as a cardiologist, this test is not invasive or painful and can be performed in less than half an hour. The test involves a vibrating device placed on the patient's chest that uses sound waves to create moving images of the heart and its chambers. The cardiologist can determine if the heart is functioning properly, or if abnormalities in its function are contributing to a patient's breathing symptoms.

A Final Word

This chapter has touched on many complex conditions that may have an asthmatic component and discusses multiple tests used in the evaluation of asthma. Despite the appearance of complexity, however, it is important to keep in mind that most cases of asthma and allergy are diagnosed using a minimum of tests. The harder part is sticking to the prescribed medical and behavioral treatments that can keep this chronic condition under control.

The Hows and Whys of Allergy And Asthma Medication

Duplicate Medication, an Expensive Problem

THIS IS CHAPTER 8, BUT IT WOULD HAVE BEEN POETIC JUSTICE IF it were chapter 11 because cost is an escalating complication for any allergy-asthma patient, and astronomical medical bills are now the number one cause of bankruptcies. Medication is expensive enough when you are getting the right ones, but too many patients often don't get what they're paying for because they're paying for more than they need, as the following illustrates.

A Fine Mess

Mrs. Smith was the mother of a 14-year-old son, Jack. When she made an appointment for an initial visit with him, I asked, as I always do, that she bring all her boy's medicines with her. She entered carrying a purse the size of a bowling bag and hauled out: albuterol, Ventolin, Proventil, Maxair, Singulair, Accolate, Flovent, Pulmicort, Serevent, Foradil, Aerobid, Theo-Dur, and Uniphyl. In addition she had the newer preparations of Advair and Symbicort. These combination products contain an anti-inflammatory and bronchodilator.

I looked at the pile on my desk. I looked at her and asked, "Mrs. Smith, do you like to cook?"

She was startled by my question. "Yes, why do you ask?"

I said, "Have you ever come across a recipe that called for oregano, basil, nutmeg, cinnamon, cloves, asafetida, cayenne, jalapeños, parsley, sage, rosemary, and thyme?"

"No. Those are all strong herbs and spices. It would be a mess."

"Precisely," I said, "and that's what you've got here. A mess."

— *Dr. Chiaramonte*

Mrs. Smith was an extreme example of fairly common type of allergy parent. In the search for relief, she never found a doctor she didn't like. What do doctors do? They prescribe medicine, and if a current medication isn't working, they prescribe something else. A new doctor will prescribe something different from the old doctor. But the Mrs. Smiths of the world won't take the hint and stop using the old ones: They use them all—or rather their children do. At best, the medication mess does no harm. And at worst?

The first thing I did was to arrange the medications into separate piles on my desk in front of Mrs. Smith:

"Pile A. These are the fast-acting bronchodilators: albuterol, Ventolin, Proventil, Maxair. In fact, the first three are really the same medication.

"Pile B. These are longer-acting bronchodilators and have a slower onset of action, but last longer: Serevent, Foradil.

"Pile C. Singulair and Accolate: These are not steroids, but counter the swelling and tissue damage to the airway lining by blocking the leukotrienes released from the mast cell along with histamine.

"Pile D. Theo-Dur and Uniphyl: These are a form of theophylline that we do not use much any more because of its narrow range of safety and effectiveness.

"Pile E. Inhaled steroids: Flovent, Pulmicort, and Aerobid. These are the best weapons we have to counter the swelling and tissue damage to the airway lining. They get a bad reputation because of the word 'steroid.' The more we use them, the more we find them to be effective and safe. But your son shouldn't be using them all at the same time.

"Pile F. Advair is a combination of Flovent and Serevent. Symbicort has as a bronchodilator Foradil and as an anti-swelling agent Pulmicort. Both do pretty much the same job. Symbicort works fast; Advair comes as a powder and may be easier to take. Both are more convenient than taking their components separately."

Mrs. Smith looked at me, a bit embarrassed. "I'm not sure that he is."

Why was I not surprised? Nor was I surprised that her son didn't seem to be getting any better.   — *Dr. Chiaramonte*

Not only was her son not getting any better, but also it is our suspicion that Mrs. Smith was paying through the nose for all that medicine. Not only are the co-payments $10 or $20 per medication, but her insurance company probably recognized the redundancies and refused to cover them all, and being a concerned parent she probably bought the others out of her own pocket. We learned that she also had "steroid phobia" and in spite of the fact that she paid for them, she wasn't as diligent in getting her son to use the best weapon we have, although when you take three different kinds, it's not so good. To make matters worse, she was embarrassed that Jack had problems using a metered-dose inhaler (MDI). This made him a good candidate for newer delivery systems such as extenders or the newer powdered inhalers. All those doctors, and he wasn't even being fully treated.

Not Like Other Chronic Conditions

Allergy and asthma are not like other conditions that require daily medication. If you are depressed, your GP can prescribe a succession of Prozac, Zoloft, Lexapro, and so on, until you find one that deals with your state of mind with the fewest disagreeable side effects. But that's just one medication at a time; you would never take them all at once.

Allergies and asthma are more complicated because usually multiple medicines *are* used simultaneously because they attack different aspects of the disease in different tissues on different timetables. The most important thing is to remember not to take two drugs concurrently that are supposed to accomplish the same end.

Running Battle

Allergy science is struggling to catch up with the things that our bodies do naturally. While we are still looking for ways to help the natural processes work better—read the chapters on environment and immunotherapy—we can't wait for breakthroughs. Short-term damage from untreated allergy can lead to long-term irreversible damage.

In the face of the resourceful, complex immune system, any "solution" is temporary or incomplete. Yesterday's cure-all becomes today's niche player.

Fortunately, as our knowledge of the mechanisms of allergy becomes more refined, medications can be used with greater specificity. We can treat the condition we want much more effectively than we used to without doing what the military refers to as "collateral damage" to other tissue. Just as carpet-bombing in warfare has given way to "smart" weapons, our modern pharmacopoeia is more precise than our old drugs.

But you have to know how to use them. Many GPs who treat allergy still fight with old weapons, and sometimes don't recognize the enemy, as this story shows. It illustrates one of the paradoxes of allergy: Acute symptoms get acute attention. Hives or shortness of breath due to asthma, for example, are allergic symptoms no one can ignore. However, minor symptoms of the same illness might get no treatment, or superficial treatment until it boils over into acute illness.

JUST A RUNNY NOSE

My father was a wonderful pediatrician, as I have already said. He was funny, empathetic with his patients, and scientifically sound. He never retired; he just kept practicing until he passed away at the age of 77. But he had a blind spot when it came to allergies. When a patient came to him with what I might recognize as allergic rhinitis, Dr. Lennie, as he was known, might say, "It's just a runny nose." This was pretty standard for his time.

— *Dr. Ehrlich*

Dr. Lennie may have thought that you can't treat every little thing—and with colds he was right. Many doctors overprescribe antibiotics for minor viral conditions that don't respond to them and weaken their efficacy for fighting bacterial infection. However, allergic rhinitis is not a cold: It is an allergic condition and a possible precursor of asthma. It results in some 9 million doctor visits a year.

What happens with minor allergic conditions, after undertreating them, is that doctors, parents, or patients themselves will overtreat them with medication directed at the overt symptoms, not the underlying condition, or the destructive inflammation that accompanies it. Because there are many different medications within each of the four or five groups we will discuss, a patient may find her medicine chest or purse filled with several brands in the same group or groups, and we often find the patient going from one to the other.

As we have explained elsewhere, the most plausible modern theory of allergy and asthma is "one airway, one disease." By treating the minor condition, you are staving off the possibility of progressive, destructive airway remodeling.

Damage, Plain as the Nose on Your Face

When allergies in general, and asthma specifically, are occurring, the process may seem complicated and mysterious because it's hidden. Except for the sight of mucus running out of your child's nose and the sounds of stuffiness or wheezing, the disease is concealed from the world. It is manifest in a private way—your child's discomfort. That will emerge through complaining, inattentiveness, acting out in school and at home, and bad grades.

Essentially, all asthma and allergies revolve around inflammation and, in the case of asthma, constriction of muscles around the bronchial airways. To more fully understand what is going on inside the patient's body, let's find an analog that is much closer to the surface. Let's find one that is as plain as the nose on your face. In fact, let's put it right on the nose on your face.

Travel back in time. It's the morning of your high school prom. You wake up and go into the bathroom. You feel something vaguely uncomfortable on your nose, and look in the mirror. To your horror, you see the last thing you need on this big day—a zit. A big, tight, red thing that's hot to the touch. You know it will never go away by tonight. Given enough time, it will cure itself: That's what the immune system does for an infection. But this one—where it is and when it happens—will permanently scar your memories of high school, and maybe even permanently scar your face.

Acne is the product of inflammation and infection, but we want to concentrate on the former. A pimple becomes red and swollen and painful and itchy; surrounding tissues become enlarged. On the skin this inflammation is uncomfortable and unsightly. When this reaction happens in a closed area like the airways of the lungs or in the nose, it prevents the vital movement of air, which can be life threatening.

If the fluid on the skin is left to dry, it becomes crusty and hard. Fluid in a closed airway dries up as you breathe and the result is a thick plug that clogs the narrow airway, sticking to the delicate tissue around it. Picture mucus left on a glass plate to dry, and then try scraping it off. None of this is pleasant to think of, but when we start to talk of the urgency of effective, timely treatment of allergies, remember this picture: This is a your child's lung on asthma.

You know how tight the skin is around that swollen pimple? Picture the muscles around your child's airways and how, when they are constricted, they will reduce your child's breathing capacity. A principle of physics says that flow rate—of air, in this case—through a tube is exponentially related to the radius of the airway. You know what happens to six lanes of highway traffic at rush hour when one lane is closed. Likewise, a small reduction in the airway size can result in a sixteenfold reduction of flow through that airway. There is very little margin, either in the nose or the lungs.

The body is well meaning. Constriction in the event of an infection has a positive side. It keeps the inflammation contained and keeps the offending matter from traveling to parts of the body where it might do more damage. Migrating inflammation can cause big time problems. There's a condition called endocarditis, for example, that sometimes occurs after dental work. If you are a fan of the TV show *NYPD Blue*, you may recall that Detective Bobby Simone died of it. An infection introduced by a puncture in his gum by the dentist ended up spreading to a heart valve.

Unfortunately, as we said in an earlier chapter, allergic inflammation travels routinely from the upper airways to the lower airways. Like endocarditis, it ends up in the place where it does the most damage.

Constriction might be useful in containing infection from a zit, but when it takes place in the lungs, it causes big problems. The lungs can't wait for the constriction to end on its own because in the meantime that delicate tissue will be damaged. To return to the prom, think of the all-time prom nightmare, the movie *Carrie*.

When the bucket of blood falls on her head Carrie realizes that she is being mistreated. The first thing she does with her telekinetic powers is to shut and lock all the doors of the gym, and with all her tormentors locked inside, all hell breaks loose. With Carrie's reactions (for our purposes, inflammation) out of control, she wreaks havoc on the enclosed gym (the lungs). The inflammatory material can't escape because all the doors are shut (airways are constricted); the fire and havoc consumes all the people (lung tissue) inside.

How does it end? In the movie, the town loses a generation of young people. In your child's lungs, the problem can be disastrous— over 5,000 people die of acute asthma every year, and there are more than 500,000 emergency room visits. Chances are it won't be fatal, but repeated episodes of inflammation take their toll.

Look at yourself in the mirror: Do you have any acne scars? Do you know anyone who had chronic acne as a teenager, whose face is now deeply pitted or pockmarked? Do you know why dermatologists recommend strict hygiene and diet regimes for severe acne patients, and prescribe them antibiotics or the medicine Accutane, which has to be discontinued months before a contemplated pregnancy? It's to spare them the agony of teenage vanity or a lifetime of mental anguish over facial disfigurement.

Do you know why we give your child a comprehensive regimen of allergy and asthma medication along with a program of lifestyle changes? It's to spare him or her a lifetime of diminished lung capacity from progressive, chronic inflammation and the continual threat of hospitalization.

What's more, this can be accomplished with very few side effects, fewer all the time. But the medication regimen must be precise, precisely observed, and regularly monitored.

Inflammation, Still Widely and Dangerously Neglected

Just to give you an idea how widely—and dangerously—treatment guidelines are ignored, consider the following.

When we were in the last stages of revising the first edition of this book in January 2003, a study was published by the GlaxoSmith-Kline, the drug company. It examined its slow-acting but long duration bronchodilator called Serevent, the brand name for salmeterol, although we suspect it could probably apply to any such medication. The study showed that people who used the drug without a cortico-steroid to control inflammation were subject to significantly greater risks of "asthma-related events"—including emergency room visits, intubation, and death—than those who used the steroids. African Americans were particularly at risk, as is the case with asthma in general. It also showed that only 50 percent of Caucasians and 38 percent of African Americans were using the steroids.

In the years since then, salmeterol has been restricted to use as an "adjuvant therapy" in patients whose asthma is not adequately controlled on inhaled corticosteroids.

This makes perfect sense when you consider the physiology of asthma. Bronchodilation relaxes muscles in the airways so that air can pass through. Inflamed adjacent tissues, however, are swollen and inflexible. Imagine filling a bicycle tire with air. The inner tube is flexible and expands. But what would happen if the tire itself were made of the same rubber that bowling balls once were made of instead of soft, flexible rubber? That flexible inner tube would wear out much more quickly.

Bronchodilators are not complete treatment for the disease called asthma. They are there to help keep the airways open by relaxing the bronchial muscles. But the surrounding tissue is under a great deal of stress and it must be treated too. Failing to treat both conditions can be fatal. In the final days before we "closed" this manuscript prior to publication, the U.S. Food and Drug Administration issued yet another warning for single-purpose long-acting bronchodilators:

"Drugs in the class of long-acting beta agonists (LABAs) should never be used alone in the treatment of asthma in children or adults. Manufacturers will be required to include this warning in the product labels of these drugs, along with taking other steps to reduce the overall use of these medications."

These new requirements are based on the FDA's analysis of clinical trials showing that use of these long-acting medicines is associated with an increased risk of severe worsening of asthma symptoms, leading to hospitalization in both children and adults and death in some patients with asthma.

More Work to Do on Educating Patients

If the whole world had read the first edition of our book, patients would dutifully take their inflammation-controlling medications as directed. Sadly, as our disappointing sales would indicate, we and our colleagues still have much more to do.

A study published in 2009 by the Asthma and Allergy Foundation of America (AAFA) called *The Asthma G.A.P. in America II: General Awareness and Perceptions* found that 97 percent of asthma patients understand that uncontrolled asthma poses serious health risks, but that 70 percent who use asthma controller medicine stop taking their medicine when their symptoms go away.

The results can be dangerous and expensive, with a high percentage of these patients reporting a significant event: 17 percent have an emergency doctor visit, 12 percent miss work, 12 percent end up in an emergency room, and 15 percent report some other serious health consequence.

Quality of Life—The Real Point of Aggressive Treatment

As the information about Serevent shows us, aggressive asthma treatment can be a matter of life and death. But the real point of aggressive allergy treatment is both far less dramatic and much more significant.

RAG JAG

A few weeks after the new school year started, 10-year-old Alfie was in my office. It was ragweed season. He was depressed and his mother was very upset because his teacher had complained that his prolonged sneezing jags were disrupting the entire class.

"What are they like?" I asked.

After rubbing the tip of his nose. "First, the tip of my nose starts to itch," he said, by now twitching his nose up and down like a rabbit. "Then I start to feel a pain inside, like someone is shoving a needle into me."

Alfie started to sneeze. One after another. Really loud. No wonder his teacher complained. I handed him a tissue. But instead of wiping his nose, he squeezed the nostrils together. Anything to stop sneezing.

"It's OK," I said. "Don't keep it in like that—it's bad for you." Finally, after he had stopped, the poor kid looked worn out.

"It hurts," he said. "And I feel numb all over."

— *Dr. Chiaramonte*

You might say, Well, it's only sneezing. But it's not. It's painful, disruptive to his schoolmates, and detrimental to his ability to pay attention in school. This is a quality of life issue for a child. A kid who can't concentrate, and distracts his classmates because of his sneezing, or, say, an asthmatic child who gives up on the more traditional, aerobic sports and looks to the ping-pong table or the bowling alley for his physical education is losing out.

DUST TO DUST

My 12-year-old patient Mordechai was preparing for his bar mitzvah when his distraught parents brought him into the office. He was adamant about not continuing his studies, which included reading extensively from the Torah, because since he started studying the scrolls he had become congested, been losing sleep, and begun snorting. Furthermore, his friends were making fun of him because he "dripped" over everything.

"I'm not going to any more studying, and that's that," he said, and that was that. Oy vey!

A detailed history revealed that he had used eight medications, but none seemed to make inroads into the problem. It became clear to me that the Torah was the source of his symptoms. Testing found him very allergic to dust mites, and as he poured over this sacred—but dusty—scroll his exposure became the issue. (Where is King Solomon when you need him?) We rapidly desensitized him to the mites (by giving him "allergy shots" or immunotherapy), placed him on a nonsedation antihistamine prior to his exposure to the Torah, and he reached the big day without a problem.   — *Dr. Ehrlich*

Relief is Not Necessarily Treatment

Everyone who has an allergic disease, from the "merely annoying" to the life-threatening, will settle at some point for short-term comfort at the expense of long-term health. Thus, someone whose nose is constantly clogged because of allergic rhinitis will snort nasal sprays like Neo-Synephrine or Afrin just to breathe through her nose again. This is an effective medicine. It contains the active ingredient *phenylephrine*, which constricts dilated blood vessels and shrinks swollen nasal passages. But it is also temporary. When it wears off, the vessels dilate again, wider than before. That's why the label says, "If symptoms persist, consult your physician." Soon you're spraying just to counteract the effect of the medicine itself (called *rhinitis medicamentosa*). And it may be very difficult to give it up. An allergist can help you. It's okay to seek temporary relief for a cold, but if the cause of congestion is an underlying allergy, it will only go away at the end of the pollen season, say, or when the molds are removed from the home, and it can come back again later.

RAW TRUTH

A 50-year-old man came to me for chronic nasal congestion. I looked up his nose with the otoscope and was appalled. His nasal passages looked like raw hamburger.

"How long have you been using Neo-Synephrine?"

"Twenty-five years."   — *Dr. Ehrlich*

Over a long period of time, that cycle of constriction and dilation wears the blood vessels out—hence the chopped-meat look. What would happen to your water pipes in your house if every time your shower got weaker you compensated by turning up the pressure of the water coming into the house, without checking the pipes themselves for leaks or blockages? Sooner or later you might have a flood. Likewise, these Neo-Synephrine addicts get nosebleeds and infections.

Neo-Synephrine and Afrin also have another complication: They are available without a prescription. Instead of the inconvenience and expense of going to a doctor, patients will choose to treat themselves. Over-the-counter drugs like these have their place in today's busy world, but they are to long-term health what a Big Mac is to a balanced diet: good for an occasional treat, but disastrous day-in, day-out.

Poor Role Model

With asthma, the dangers are even greater. Who hasn't heard of Primatene? This is the oldest asthma inhaler. It has been advertised on television and the radio for decades, and it is currently a prominent sponsor of after-midnight programming, complete with celebrity endorsers. But do these athletes actually use the stuff, assuming they have asthma? Not if their team physicians have anything to do with it, because the active ingredients don't just affect the lungs, they stimulate the heart. They have both beta-2, which works on the lungs, and beta-1, which works on the heart, whereas the most common rescue inhaler we use, albuterol, is specific for the lungs. As urban pediatric allergists, this specific form of self-medication worries us a great deal.

ASTHMA CORRIDOR

A few years ago, I was consulting with a group in Hunts Point in the Bronx, a poor, substantially Puerto Rican neighborhood in what we call a high-asthma corridor. I walked past a playground and saw a number of small children playing with Primatene inhalers.

I asked our program coordinator if he knew why this was.

He answered, "Doctor, it's because it's the easiest and cheapest way for their parents to deal with their asthma. They give them the inhaler and send them to school so they can go to work." — *Dr. Ehrlich*

Trailing-Edge Medicine

The primacy of Primatene in a poor neighborhood should surprise no one. If an upper-middle class person walks through a poor neighborhood, they will see things that have long since disappeared from their own environs: Billboards that advertise menthol cigarettes, malt liquor, and brandy are regular sights. Quick fixes to get people over life's big problems.

The same is true with some trailing-edge medications—medications whose limitations are well known but are so cheap to produce that it's still worth it to the manufacturers to keep them on the market.

Still, the fact that a drug is an "oldie" does not mean it is obsolete. For example, *pseudoephedrine*, sold as Sudafed, is pretty much it when you need a decongestant, and it works. (This is the active ingredient of homebrew methamphetamine, after all, stolen straight from the drug-store shelves.)

When you see the letter D after a drug name, it means there's pseudoephedrine in it. But beware: When you give a time-release drug with a decongestant in it to a child, you are putting a very large dose of a strong stimulant into her body. Is "time release" really as controlled as we're supposed to think?

Other effective older medications are the first-generation anti-histamines, which are still very useful at times and since they are available in generic form, they are both cheaper and easier to find in an emergency than many other drugs. Furthermore, we are in the business of doing the best for our patients. We will use these drugs in our practice if they work.

Some older drugs have their drawbacks; so do new ones for that matter. Older antihistamines, nonprescription Benadryl and Chlor-Trimeton, and prescription Atarax—hydroxyzine—cross the brain-blood barrier, for example, which makes you drowsy. The sedative

---

BENADRYL INADVERTENTLY SAVES A LIFE

How many times does a drug save a life not because it worked but because it of its side effects? I had a patient whose allergies plagued her badly in summer and fall of 2001. A recent college graduate, she was supposed to start a new job soon. Nothing I gave her helped, and her mother called frequently to let me know. The latest drug I gave her was Zyrtec. For a time, I didn't hear from them. Then one day, she called again to make an appointment for her daughter.

I looked at the chart and asked Mom, "How's the Zyrtec working?"

She answered, "It's not. She took Benadryl, and it saved her life."

On the morning the daughter was supposed to start her new job, Mom said, "She called me at 7:00 a.m. and told me how miserable she was because the Benadryl made her so tired. Since I knew her boss, I told her, 'If you feel that bad, stay home, and you'll start next week instead.'"

Her new office was on the 103rd floor of the World Trade Center, and her scheduled first day was September 11, 2001.

— *Dr. Ehrlich*

---

effects of Benadryl are so well known, in fact, that the comic crime novelist Carl Hiassen had a villain load a bowl of fish chowder with twenty doses for her husband to eat before he went scuba diving. He nodded off and drowned. But that doesn't mean it's a bad drug, if used as directed.

Money, Money, Money

There's no question that trailing-edge medications provide relief. They work within minutes or hours, whereas immunotherapy takes months. But then what? You keep paying for years. Absent health insurance, an effective prescription drug can cost $100–$150 a month, and an effective asthma steroid spray may cost $200 a month. With a $10-plus co-payment per prescription, a combination of drugs begins to add up.

As second-generation antihistamines like Claritin and Zyrtec roll off prescription, the cost structure has been shaken up, but generic versions of these drugs still run about 50 cents per pill.

When we wrote the original version of this book, we were looking forward to seeing if the generic versions of previously prescription drugs would shake up insurance reimbursement. Would insurers decline to cover prescription drugs, thus taking valuable weapons out of the hands of doctors? In fact, the situation is even more ominous than that. At least one major self-insuring union in New York, which really should know better, categorically will not cover anything to do with allergies: no meds, no immunotherapy, nothing. They have decided that they can save a lot of money by not covering allergies, their members be damned.

If anyone doubts the importance of avoidance and immuno-therapy as primary tools in treatment, put dollar signs on long-term drug costs. Immunotherapy, by contrast, has front-loaded costs and considerable effort attached to it, but in the long run is highly benefi-cial with little or no effort.

New Drugs Get Old Very Quickly

With the science of allergy as dynamic as it is, the time between today's new breakthrough and tomorrow's trailing edge become shorter and shorter.

To understand why drugs age so quickly, it helps to know how clinical trials are conducted. There are three phases to an FDA trial:

Phase One: You have to prove that the drug is not lethal.

Phase Two: You prove it is effective for the indicated condition.

Phase Three: You pay doctors to administer it to 5,000 or 10,000 patients to ascertain wider effectiveness and side effects. After phase three, if the benefits outweigh the problems by a convincing degree, you can release it. Martha Stewart's legal woes over insider trading stemmed from early notification that the government was dissatisfied with a phase three result, which meant that the drug wouldn't go on the market and thus make shareholders rich.

Yet, even after phase three, a drug must prove itself. Side effects that never showed up in clinical trials will show up in practice, even some that we might call "false negatives." For example, there was a good drug called Seldane that was potentially lethal in some when used in combination with certain other medications. This effect never showed up in controlled trials because trials involve comprehensive medical history, including other drugs, so certain combinations were disallowed. In practice, this precaution isn't usually taken. So we lost an effective drug because of insufficiently conscientious medical practice.

Even without such dire outcomes, the magnitude of the leap from trial to prescription will involve complications. There's a big difference between 5,000–10,000 patients and the hundreds of thousands who will get the drug after its release. The drug may be ineffective or may have bad side effects for a statistically insignificant number of people in a trial, but even if it's just one percent, when 100,000 people are taking it, that leaves 1,000 who need something else. For those people, the new miracle drug is no miracle at all. And over a period of time, its shortcomings are likely to become magnified. Every time referrals to our offices dry up from one doctor or another, it usually coincides with some new drug release, but over time, new patients start to trickle in as the miracle starts to wear off.

This was certainly the case with a drug called Singulair, which pediatricians loved because it could be taken orally—you sometimes have to hold a kid down to teach him to use an inhaler—and because it had no steroids. But while a useful drug, its great wave of popularity crested as it showed its limitations; it was not the panacea it first appeared to be. Many patients still needed the combination of treatments allergists offer.

Leading-Edge Medication

One of the dreams of allergists is the idea of an "anti-IgE" medication, one that would block the action of the antibody IgE present in the patient from reacting with the offending allergens and so setting off an allergic response. The experimental drug TNX-901, which we noted in our food allergy chapter for its prophylactic use against peanut allergy, was supposed to be such a drug. However, as we mentioned, it was discontinued.

An Allergist's Medication Strategy

The way the two of us look at it, there are no wonder drugs, even temporary ones. Nothing will work forever in all people. We would like to help our patients get to the point where their bodies can do more of the work themselves through immunotherapy, or at the very least reduce exposure to the allergens through lifestyle changes, thereby minimizing the occurrence of disease with accompanying inflammation.

However, we know that the first challenge is just to get the thing under control.

The first major advantage we offer is that we are up on the latest medications targeted at specific conditions. We read the literature on trials, we go to the meetings where these drugs are presented, and we talk with the people at the companies that produce them. So chances are we have the latest weapons in our arsenal, whereas a busy GP, who has to keep up with developments in a broad array of specialties, won't.

Second of all, because we know the strengths and weaknesses of the full allergy pharmacopoeia, we recognize that there are certain trailing-edge medications that still have their uses for limited purposes.

For example, a new patient who comes to us who is wary of inhaled steroids and strong laboratory-created medications might be persuaded to use *cromolyn sodium* (known as NasalCrom or Opticrom), which you will read about in greater detail later on. A nebulizer version of this called Intal has now been discontinued, although we wish someone would bring it back.

Cromolyn sodium, for all its Chemistry 101 sound, is derived from an Egyptian root, and has probably been used in some form for medical purposes since before Moses was pulled from the bulrushes. We used to recommend the inhaled form as a kind of training inhalant. After our patients got accustomed to feeling better, we would work on a stronger and more effective program of modern targeted pharmaceuticals. Again, economics were the enemy.

One of the problems with cromolyn sodium was that you had to take it fairly often. This is also the case with the nasal spray. The pain-in-the-neck factor is an important consideration in allergy and asthma treatment. If taking medication is annoying, people stop using it when they feel better. Disease and inflammation will return.

The pain-in-the-neck factor applies not just to the number of times our patients must use the medication but how many medications they take. It is very basic to our approach that we try to keep the number of medicines down. While a combination of medicines may work very effectively together, we don't want medication fatigue to set in. The more fed up patients get with the regimen, the less likely they are to stick to the program, and thus miss out on effective treatment.

Another very popular asthma medicine, a leukotriene receptor antagonist called Accolate, illustrates another form of pain-in-the-neck factor, particularly for use in children. Namely, it had to be taken twice a day, but hours before and after meals. You can't wake a child up hours before breakfast every day to give him a drug or keep him up for hours after dinner. And are you going to trust your child to take the medicine in the middle of her morning at school, or in midafternoon? Good luck. Even adults have trouble with this restriction. So just remember, every time something comes on the market as the greatest thing since sliced bread, sooner or later it will get stale.

Niche Medicines

Cromolyn sodium is also a perfect example of a niche medicine that can be used tactically for certain situations. One of the things that make it incredibly useful as a niche medicine is that it is incredibly safe and side effect–free. The other is that it works to stave off allergic reactions when taken before and even during high exposure to allergens.

For example, if your child is allergic to cats and you're going to visit Aunt Rachel with her beloved calico cat Rambo for the weekend, your child might start puffing cromolyn sodium on Friday.

Off-Label Uses

Another advantage of the allergist's approach to using medications is that we are aware of the chemistry behind a particular medicine and thus might use it in ways that are not enumerated in the *Physicians' Desk Reference* (PDR) or on the literature from the manufacturer.

For example, that pain-in-the-neck medicine Accolate, which is an anti-leukotriene, might be useful situationally for hives without the long-term discipline necessary when using it for asthma. If you recall from our chapter on the mechanics of allergy, leukotrienes are released by cells after the first assault of histamines, and hives are one of the products of leukotrienes. Thus, a short course of anti-leukotrienes can combat the itching of hives, their inflammatory effect, and the potential for scarring that not only ensues from the eruption itself but from a child's overpowering urge to scratch.

One problem with off-label uses of drugs is that they may not be reimbursable for these secondary purposes. They must be tested and approved for each condition. The asthma drug Xolair, which we mention above, is expected to be effective for peanut allergy, but because its pending approval is only for asthma, use for peanuts would not be covered by insurance.

Add-On Medications

A class of drugs considered partially anti-inflammatory are called leukotriene antagonists. These medications, such as montelukast

(Singulair), zafirlukast (Accolate), and zileuton (Zyflo), work against one variety of inflammation-causing substances that increase in children with exercise- and allergy-induced asthma. Hence, they are often added to inhaled corticosteroids when these factors are identified as triggers in individual cases. They are not recommended for use as the only anti-inflammatory drug for asthma treatment because they block only one aspect of inflammation, whereas corticosteroids treat the inflammation that results from all these chemical effects, not just one of them.

Another variety of add-on controller medications is the long-acting bronchodilators, such as the above-mentioned salmeterol. They reportedly help reduce the dose of inhaled corticosteroid needed to maintain control. They also help reduce nighttime flares and are of benefit in exercise-induced asthma.

A combination of salmeterol and fluticasone known as Advair is available in dry-powder formulation that is inhaled using a Diskus device. It is available in different strengths, but only the corticosteroid strength changes, not the salmeterol. Its ease of use (one inhalation twice daily) favors good compliance, however the fixed combination makes flexibility more difficult when more steroids are needed to treat acute asthma flares. This medication is not approved for children under the age of 12. We must emphasize that Advair is *not* a remedy for acute asthma.

Strategic Thinking

Asthma and allergy medications are constantly being improved. However, while they get better at what they do, *what* they do basically remains the same. Some block the release of mediators, both fast acting and slow acting, some reverse physical processes such as swelling, and some fight inflammation. This is a more complex version of what we have always done: When we started out in this field we dealt with these problems in broad strokes—using systemic antihistamines, adrenaline, and steroids. Now the drugs are more specific in how they are delivered and where they work in the body. We also have a more sophisticated knowledge of how the disease travels in the body and how it progresses. One airway, one disease. The new drugs allow us to block the progress of each incident before it comes to reside in the most vulnerable part of the body, the lungs.

What is missing from most medication regimens is a strategy based on this progression. Simply put, some medicines deal with muscle constriction or swelling, some interrupt the progress of the attack, and some reduce inflammation. With all these intricacies, we need to keep our medications straight. Moreover, we have to avoid duplication, as in the case of Mrs. Smith, who never met a doctor she didn't like enough to fill a prescription. The only ones who benefit from that situation are the companies that make each individual drug. Her insurance companies, the doctors themselves, her bank account, and particularly her son, were all net losers.

A good medication strategy would target the discrete allergic mechanisms with the best possible medication. Mrs. Smith's son's asthma was not only overseasoned but baked, fried, and boiled.

Compliance—A Crucial Part of Medication Strategy

Of course, the best regimen of drugs won't do any good at all if they are not taken as directed, which is what we call in medicine "compliance" (which we will discuss more fully in our chapter on alternative medicine). And Mrs. Smith's son was clearly not in compliance. There were a number of problems. First of all, taking all those medicines as directed would obviously be a pain in the neck. What 14-year-old would put up with it? Second, with all those medicines, some of which provided immediate relief and some of which treated the underlying condition, Jack tended to use the ones that provided relief as they were needed and ignore the rest—a common tendency and a destructive one because, as you will recall from Asthma Basics, some of the worst damage is done when symptoms are not obvious.

Finally, and this is one where Mrs. Smith is clearly an enabler, because she is steroid-phobic, she soft-peddles the use of steroids when in fact they are all-important.

For some children, good compliance is simply a matter of their own comfort. Yanicka Faustin of Brooklyn, New York, takes her medicine regularly because she finds the sensation of albuterol working its way through her lungs uncomfortable if she doesn't use it just right. For others, the speedy feeling of the albuterol can be disturbing.

Routine—An Important Reinforcer of Compliance

Taking daily medication requires commitment. When the medication is working, it's easy to forget that you are prone to sickness. To help reinforce that commitment, it helps to have a routine. An antidepressant might be kept next to your coffee maker in the morning to remind you that one is as much a part of getting started in the morning as the other. A cholesterol drug might be kept next to the bread that will make the toast on which you will slather jelly instead of butter.

With allergies and asthma, routine is harder to establish, especially for children. Essentially, you have to establish two routines: one for yourself and one for the child. If the child is asymptomatic, you have to remind yourself to remind her to take her medications. This problem is compounded by the fact that the medication may vary from time to time based on variances in peak flow, which might call for some change in the regimen. One of the benefits of peak flow monitoring is that it can be done regularly regardless of symptoms. If your peak flow is in the green zone every day, that doesn't mean it shouldn't be done because you never know.

The Wrong Words

Mark Twain is known for saying, "The difference between the right word and the almost right word is the difference between lightning and lightning bug." With asthma, the difference between the right word and the almost right word may be health or illness.

Nancy Sander, founder of Allergy & Asthma Network Mothers of Asthmatics (AANMA), was once on an airplane and struck up a conversation with a woman who worked for Planned Parenthood who described herself as a "noncompliant asthmatic." Upon further questioning, she hauled a set of medicines out of her purse and identified one as her "controller," one as her "reliever," one as her "preventer," and one as her "rescuer." She had stopped taking the first three and every time she started to wheeze, she took her "rescuer"—the powerful drug albuterol. Nancy asked the woman, "Isn't it better that your clients practice conscientious birth control rather than have abortions for unwanted pregnancies?" The startled woman answered, "Of course." Nancy's reaction was, "Then why do you treat your asthma with the most drastic remedy instead of keeping the worst symptoms from happening in the first place." Sheepishly, the woman answered, "Because I can never keep straight which one is supposed to do what."

Another literary reference, the last for a while we promise:

Ernest Hemingway was supposedly asked what a writer should do with the first draft of a novel. He said, "First go through and cross out all the adjectives." The theory is that strong nouns don't need modifiers. The same is true with asthma medication. Adjectives commonly used to describe medication are frequently ambiguous.

The Big Offenders Are "Controller," "Reliever," "Preventer," and "Rescue"

The primary "rescue" medication, the bronchodilator albuterol, does open up constricted airways in emergencies, but it also controls wheezing and prevents attacks if taken before exercise. Which heading does it ultimately fall under? Because they affect so many phases of asthma, bronchodilators end up as the default medications for any and all purposes. It becomes the lowest common denominator of asthma treatment instead of a true emergency medicine. This can't be good for you because it means that not only is chronic, low-level inflammation permitted to take place, but also that you are routinely taking hits of a powerful stimulant as well.

Just as ambiguous is a "preventer" medicine such as a corticosteroid, which also provides relief, controls inflammation, and so on.

Nancy points out that when asthmatics are experiencing symptoms, they don't bother to sort out whether the symptoms should be classified as requiring control, relief, prevention, or rescue. They want something that works, and what always works is their bronchodilator, whether that it is the appropriate medication or not. They don't think about which of the four things the medicine is supposed to do, they act on their perception of what is happening to them, and they reflexively reach for the wrong one. "Is this mild wheezing or are my lungs about to seize up? Better not take any chances."

The AANMA recommends the Hemingway approach: Get rid of the adjectives. This is what your authors believe, too. We don't use those adjectives. Rather, it is better, even for children who are beginning to take control (that's the noun form, not the adjective) of their own medication, to learn the names of each medicine and its uses.

If you go back to the beginning of this book, you'll realize that the initial approach in the treatment of any of the allergic diseases, be it allergic rhinitis, eczema, urticaria (hives), conjunctivitis (inflammation of the eyelids), asthma, or food allergies, is to avoid the offender or the "thing" that initiates the problem to begin with. To that end, nothing is easier to treat by avoidance than food allergies. If kumquats cause hives, avoid kumquats. Milk—now there it gets more difficult. Children should drink milk, and it appears hidden in lots of foods.

If your 4-year-old who is allergic around a cat is going to Aunt Rachel's where there is a cat, a medication to prevent the release of all those mast cell mediators (cromolyn) or one that will block the mediators' effects (an antihistamine) on the tissues (skin, nose, lungs, gastrointestinal tract, or all of them) must be given prior to the cat exposure. If more potent medications are required for prevention, we've got them. If symptoms occur in spite of the use of these medications, then the tissue reactions (hives, rhinitis, wheezing, nausea, and vomiting, or all of them) must be reversed.

Green, Yellow, and Red Days

The crux of any asthma medication regimen is a color-coded "Asthma Action Plan." This is developed individually for patients and is based on what their personal best peak flow meter reading is and what medications they are currently on. A traffic light is used as the framework for the asthma action plan. The green zone is "good" and the medications are only the maintenance medicines. The peak flow readings are 80–100 percent of the personal best. The yellow zone means to "slow down (not speed up)" because their peak flow readings are dropping. The numbers range between 50–80 percent of their personal best. At this time additional medications such as a bronchodilator and additional inhaled corticosteroids are added to help improve the numbers. If the readings do not improve or continue to get worse, the person needs to be evaluated and treated by their physician. If the peak flow readings drop into the red zone, this is called the "danger" zone. This is when the readings are less than 50 percent of their personal best. At this time nebulized broncho-dilators or a metered-dose inhaler bronchodilator are often used. The individual is also instructed to seek treatment immediately. The purpose of this plan is to assist the patients to feel comfortable managing their asthma and have more control over their illness. Information about the Asthma Action Plan and the medications used may be found online from Asthma & Allergy Network Mothers of Asthmatics at www.aanma.org and from Dr. Tom Plaut's Pedi-press at www.pedipress.com.

Ease of Use

It is important to remember that the effectiveness of any medi-cation is in part determined by proper use. When a metered-dose inhaler is used for asthma, the medication is released at a very high speed (60–80 miles per hour). This makes it diffi-cult to coordinate the release of the puff at the same time as the inhalation of breath. Further, placing the inhaler in the mouth can produce greater side effects from the drug being absorbed through the mouth into the bloodstream. This is the case with the MDI pirbuterol (Maxair Autohaler), which is activated auto-matically by placing the device in the mouth and taking in a deep breath.

Thus, drug delivery to the airways is important. A device called a holding chamber greatly enhances proper use of most inhalers. As most rescue inhalers require two puffs, it is essential to wait a minimum of two minutes before the second puff. This allows time for the first puff to open up the airways so that the second puff gets down even further into the smaller airways.

A note of caution, however: During a severe attack your child may not be able to breathe in deeply enough to activate the inhaler.

Regarding the issue of proper use, it is essential that nebulizer treatments for infants and small children be done with a mask over the mouth and nose. Using a mouthpiece with closed lips is also acceptable for older children and adults. Blow-by technique (holding the tube in front of the mouth and nose) does not allow for proper delivery of the nebulized medication.

Guidelines or Recipe?

We have mentioned the problem of too many physicians failing to follow treatment guidelines. In the case of something like bronchodilators being used without steroids, these guidelines should be etched in stone. However, there is no cookie-cutter approach to allergy or asthma treatment. Most medications have strengths and weaknesses and can be effectively used alone or in combination. Some work for some people and not for others. Given the level of compliance issues we have talked about, even very good drugs end up not fulfilling their potential. Ultimately, each child's allergies and asthma are unique, and each program of treatment is a custom product. The ultimate answer may be a surprise, as the following story shows.

TRIAL AND ERROR

Jonny is a 3-year-old boy with bronchial asthma and allergic rhinitis whose nocturnal cough had been a problem for a year or so prior to his evaluation in our office. He was under the care of a fine pediatrician and a superb alternative-care doctor who instituted a program of allergen avoidance with modest success.

Our initial work-up found him to have a stuffy nose and coughing that kept him and his parents up night after night. A succession of antihistamines, including Allegra, Claritin, and Zyrtec, along with some over-the-counter preparations, made only a slight difference.

At one point it was apparent that Jonny also had problems with bronchial asthma (no wheezing, but coughing). I prescribed a nebulizer, added Proventil, and we were in business, or so I thought. He responded somewhat, but the cough still was a problem, and no one was getting any rest. An inhaled steroid (Pulmicort Respules) was added, and I thought we were home free. No way.

While he seemed to have a clear chest with no rapid breathing or wheezing, and his cough became *(continued on next page)*

---

intermittent, he still had coughing at night, and his parents still were exhausted. Back to the office and another exam, and I found the answer … or did I? Another look into Jonny's nose revealed a thick, gelatinous mess that none of his doctors, including me, had seen before, but certainly gave me a reason to think that this cough was really from a postnasal drip. He had been on a succession of antihistamine-decongestant combinations, but they weren't doing the job. All contained pseudoephedrine as the decongestant, but it was apparent that the oral medications were not doing their jobs.

All right, let's go to the anatomical source of the problem and try a nasal steroid. While Rhinocort Aqua and Nasacort AQ were two of many available, I opted for one most often used in children, Nasonex. Now Jonny had used some OTC (over-the-counter) preparation in the past, including NasalCrom, and was not crazy about putting anything up his nose, but I figured that Nasonex would go right to the root of the problem. So what happened? You guessed it: He was still coughing, although his chest still sounded fine.

At this point I began to think, "Well, it's a stuffy nose, and his asthma *is*, after all, under control." Maybe we should give it a rest. Then I thought about the quality of life issues:

- He was up half the night and worn out the next day.
- He was a basket case at preschool.
- His apartment-house neighbors were *kvetching* (complaining) that he was keeping them up.
- His parents were exhausted, and their work was suffering.

We had tried a mast cell stabilizer (NasalCrom), a bronchodilator (Proventil), antihistamines (Zyrtec, Allegra, and Claritin), an inhaled steroid (Pulmicort), decongestants (pseudoephedrine with and without antihistamine), and some *of* the old stand-bys such as Neo-Synephrine Nasal Spray (also a decongestant). Quite a shopping basket. A modicum of relief was achieved, however, when I thought about what my good Ear-Nose-and-Throat colleagues had taught me and realized that what Jonny's nose needed was a good cleaning. Recognizing the effects of *(continued on next page)* the nose rinsing with a hypertonic saline (2%–3% salt) solution such as SaltAire, I prevailed upon Jonny's parents to give it a try. (Remember: Jonny, like most children at that age, doesn't like "stuff" up his nose.) I would like to say that the SaltAire with subsequent Nasonex and Pulmicort Respules is doing the trick, but let's leave it that it is a "work in progress."

The point in presenting Jonny (and I want to thank his parents for allowing me to do so) is that caring for the allergic/asthmatic child involves understanding the cause of the symptoms, trials of medications, and the availability of the physician and his or her assistant to fine-tune the treatment, never forgetting quality of life issues. The pediatrician and the specialist and their staff need to work with them in mind.

— *Dr. Ehrlich*

CHAPTER 9

Immunotherapy:
Strengths and Weaknesses

WHEN YOU CONSIDER THE COMPLEX ARRAY OF WEAPONS THE immune system has in its arsenal and the strategic and tactical capabilities displayed in their deployment, you might think that the Military War College should study immunology. Furthermore, when you consider that allergies represent an ancient mechanism that has survived thousands of years of human experience and emerges when certain conditions are met, there does seem to be a kind of memory comparable to anything we have in our brains. However, as we have pointed out, many of these allergic "troops" and "weapons" have had no mission for hundreds of years but they suddenly go into action against otherwise-harmless invaders. The ideal would be to "retrain" these renegade troops not to attack. That is the purpose behind immunotherapy.

Who likes to get stuck with a needle? Who likes to watch their children get a shot?

The answers to these questions are "no one" and "no one." Anyone who answers "I do" has problems that go well beyond allergies. Yet, obnoxious as they can be, allergy injections are often—not always—the best long-term treatment for allergies, with emphasis on *often* and *long-term*. This effectiveness leads to the patient ultimately becoming more tolerant of them.

Allergy shots—a.k.a. allergen immunotherapy, specific allergen immunotherapy, hyposensitization, or desensitization—would seem like a kind of miracle treatment, a kind of slow-motion inoculation that eliminates the need for a kid to take a pharmacy of medications or be overly careful about where she goes and when. Who knows? She might even be able to clean up her room without sneezing—but don't hold your breath.

Small amounts of the material she has reacted to in diagnostic skin tests are injected into her arm with a small, *almost* painless needle. A reaction, something like a mosquito bite, may appear, although she should remain at the doctor's office for at least half an hour to monitor the severity of the reaction.

When they work, the shots are a tremendous relief not only from the symptoms of allergy but also from the other precautions we ask our children to take. They're not a panacea, however. They certainly shouldn't be done for very mild allergies; the treatment could be worse—or at least more annoying, time consuming, and expensive—than the disease. For children with really serious asthma or who are very allergic, this treatment can be beneficial but also slightly risky. Experienced allergists can really prove their worth by treating these children. There is a real question as to whether immunotherapy should be attempted before the age of 5. An allergist will make a decision based on how sick the child is and after conferring with the child's pediatrician and parents.

How They Work

There's nothing new about allergy shots. They have been used to treat allergies and asthma for nearly a century. The course of shots begins with small doses—a fraction of a unit—that are gradually increased until they reach a maximum or a maintenance dose—1,000 to 5,000 units. As the dose rises, patients start to feel better. The length of treatment, dosage, and intervals between shots vary from patient to patient depending on the clinical response.

Two Kinds of Immunotherapy

There are two kinds of allergy shots, one of which we will discuss now because it is in common use, and a second that we will hold until the end of the chapter because it is experimental, although very promising. Another new development doesn't involve needles at all, but is also in the development phase, at least in this country. We will also discuss that at the end of the chapter.

Enriquez was a 6-year-old boy who had suffered severe milk allergy and eczema almost from birth. From 2 to 4 years of age he was hospitalized five times for severe asthma. The pediatrician ordered a nebulizer with bronchodilators and inhaled steroids to be used four times a day at home. Several short courses of oral steroids were required to prevent hospitalization. The wheezing continued almost daily; Enriquez's growth began to lag.

The pediatrician ordered a total allergic antibody test (IgE) and RASTs on the boy. Everything came back extremely positive. Enriquez had almost ten times the normal amount of allergic antibodies. He reacted to many things in the environment. A program to remove allergens was begun. The cat was given away; dust control was begun in Enriquez's bedroom. These measures helped, but not enough to prevent trips to the hospital altogether. Although he had little experience with immunotherapy, the pediatrician felt forced to try a series of allergy shots on Enriquez. With the first injections, Enriquez became ill within minutes and required an injection of epinephrine to treat the reaction.

The mother persisted in looking for relief. She visited a pediatric allergist who conducted another round of skin tests. Enriquez reacted to the smallest amount of allergen. The allergist began injecting Enriquez with one allergen at a time, at minute dosage levels: one-hundredth to one-thousandth the levels that the pediatrician had been giving. Encountering no bad reaction, the allergist slowly increased the dosages over the next several months. He would delay the increases if a large local reaction appeared. After seven months of treatment, wheezing began to subside; at nine months he stopped wheezing completely; at twelve months the asthma medications were reduced, and later were eliminated completely. After two years Enriquez was a new boy. He was receiving allergy shots every two to three weeks with no additional medications, and he had no active asthma. His growth rate returned to normal, and he caught up with his age group. If this holds up, within a few more years Enriquez can stop the shots and will do well for a long time.

— *Dr. Chiaramonte*

WHAT IMMUNOTHERAPY ISN'T

The principle of immunotherapy as stated above sounds simple enough, but it must be done carefully. What passes for immunotherapy in the hands of inexperienced doctors and patients can be bizarre and would be amusing if it weren't potentially so dangerous.

When I was in the navy, a sailor came to me with a long list of allergies he had been diagnosed with that included foods, pollens, and Aqua Velva aftershave lotion. Then he showed me the serum his doctor had prepared. It had a strange blue color. I was so intrigued by the color that I asked what it had in it.

"Weren't you listening?" he snapped—allergy patients are sometimes massively self-absorbed, same as the rest of us. "I told you what I was allergic to."

I said, "I must confess that I have never seen allergy vaccine this color." Then it dawned on me. "Aqua Velva?" I asked. He nodded his head smugly. Getting him to cease using that serum was not easy. Once people place faith in a treatment or a doctor, they are reluctant to give it up. I convinced him that while shooting aftershave lotion containing alcohol and other chemicals directly into his system might not damage him greatly, it was not Aqua Velva that he was allergic to, it was a chemical in it, and one, moreover, that should respond to immunotherapy. (See list below.)

All allergies, and all treatments, are not created equal.

Another winner I met was a woman who would start to sneeze when she worked with the Xerox machine in her office. So her doctor would make her hold an open paper bag over the machine to "collect the fumes," seal it, and run it to his office where he would withdraw the air with a syringe and inject it into a vial of saline solution, shake it up, then inject her with the saline. This is allergy treatment by way of homeopathy. It is bogus, but costly, and probably reimbursable by insurance if the doctor is creative in his coding. While the injections themselves may have been harmless, if they were keeping her from seeking authentic treatment for an authentic condition, they were damaging her health by omission.

— *Dr. Ehrlich*

The first kind of immunotherapy is the 100-year-old allergy vaccine whose use we just observed in action in Enriquez's story. It contains allergens and stimulates immune cells to produce an IgG protective antibody that competes with the reaction of IgE on the mast cell. We believe that over time, levels of IgE to the offending allergen fall as IgE response diminishes and the benign IgG antibody increases. To return to our military metaphor, this would be the equivalent of IgG special operations fighters supporting local resistance fighters to attack the destructive IgE regular troops over a long period of time until the number of IgE troops can't be replenished and the good guys control the terrain.

For example, in the case of ragweed, a common cause of hay fever in the fall, a vaccine is injected in small amounts and gradually increased. The immune cells make antibodies to ragweed.

When ragweed enters the body through the airways these new blocking antibodies compete with the IgE and help the body dispose of the allergen uneventfully. The allergic IgE antibodies on the mast cells don't have a chance to cause allergic symptoms. In time the whole immune system undergoes a shift from making the allergy-producing IgE antibodies, to IgG antibodies that do not cause allergic reaction. In fact the immune system moves to a nonallergic type. This is why you may remain well for years after allergy shots stop.

How Often Do You Have to Put Up With It?

At the beginning, injections are usually given once or twice a week, although sometimes injection rates are accelerated and the beginnings of immunity can be accomplished in a matter of weeks, days, or even hours. This is called rush immunotherapy and it is not for everyone.

Recent research on grass pollen indicates that at least three years are necessary to produce the anti-allergic state, and that the benefits will last three or more years after the injections stop. The timetable may be different for other allergens and more complex allergies.

After a few months, the intervals between shots may increase to every two weeks and eventually to once a month—no small consideration for children and their parents and their busy schedules.

WHAT'S THE HURRY?

Rapid immunotherapy is not for everyone. There's always a danger of a severe response from the rapid increase of dosage levels so the gradual build up over a period of months is generally more desirable. However, sometimes there's a pressing need for speed.

We had a small girl in the hospital with subacute bacterial endocarditis, a severe infection inside her heart. This is best treated with high dosages of penicillin, but the pediatrician called us because she had had a strong allergic reaction to penicillin in the past. Skin testing confirmed penicillin allergy. We began to give her thousandths-of-a-unit of penicillin by injection and every twenty minutes doubled the dose while we sat by the bedside ready to treat any bad allergic reactions. None occurred and many hours later she received a full dose of penicillin with no bad effects. Our job was done: As long as there were no breaks in treatment, she could safely receive her penicillin. Once the treatment was completed, however, her allergy to penicillin returned in a matter of weeks.

This was an example of rush immunotherapy.　　*— Dr. Ehrlich*

Sometimes, there's no emergency, but an accelerated course of immunotherapy is still necessary. A teenaged boy named Bill was saving for college by cutting lawns. He came to us in April because the previous summer he had a severe allergic reaction to yellow jacket stings and he wanted to know what could be done for him by July, when the yellow jackets come out. How could we protect Bill by July? We had him come to our office two days a week with a day in between. We gave three increasing dosages twenty minutes apart each of those days. It took only six weeks to reach maintenance dose—full protection once a month.

This was modified rush immunotherapy.　　*— Dr Chiaramonte*

How Well Does It Work for Asthma?

When immunotherapy was first developed, asthma treatment was nowhere near as effective as it is now. The only effective way to treat an acute asthma attack was an injection of adrenaline, which relaxes the smooth muscles in the airwaves and allows the patient to breathe. However, this does nothing to rid the lungs of mucus or reduce inflammation, which, as we have already explained, constitutes the long-term threat to the patient's health.

Allergy shots represented a great leap forward for some asthma patients. However, some of them failed to respond as favorably to immunotherapy for allergens like molds and cockroaches as they did to treatment for hay fever. Questions remain about the limits of immunotherapy, although there are signs of progress as we refine the injectable allergens.

A conference in 2000 at the Cooke Institute of Allergy in New York arrived at a consensus on immunotherapy for asthma:

1. Specific allergen immunotherapy (allergy shots) has been shown, through documentation of well-controlled studies, to be effective for the treatment of allergic asthma.

2. There is emerging evidence that allergen immunotherapy can be an effective means of preventing the onset of asthma in children with allergic rhinitis. Specific allergen immunotherapy should be considered as a mode of therapy in patients with disorders that predispose to asthma, such as hay fever, after appropriate diagnosis.

3. Environmental control, appropriate use of pharmacotherapy, and allergen immunotherapy are all treatment modalities to be carefully considered with respect to therapeutic intervention for the patient with allergic respiratory disease.

These findings echoed earlier research that showed immunotherapy to be effective for stinging insect allergy as well as allergic rhinitis-conjunctivitis and allergic asthma.

But while patients with mild to moderate asthma clearly benefit from allergy shots if the asthma is triggered by allergies, severe asthmatics who have suffered from airway remodeling—permanent changes in their lungs—may benefit from immunotherapy to a limited degree. Our priority is to control inflammation, and thus stave off further damage. Some doctors—and patients and patients' parents for that matter—are so wary of using steroids that they will try treatments that are marginally promising. They must understand that the inflammation is the real villain here, not the dreaded S-word.

ALLERGY VACCINES COMMONLY USED IN TESTING AND/OR IMMUNOTHERAPY

Dust mites	Pokeweed	Elm
Household Pets	**Grasses**	Maple
Cats	Rye	Sycamore
Dogs	Bluegrass	**Molds**
Other Animals	Fescue	Alternaria
Horses	Orchard	Cladosporium
Rabbits	Sweet vernal	Aspergillus
Mice	Junegrass	Penicillium
Rats	Timothy	Other molds
Insect Venoms	Bermuda	**Foods**
Honey bees	Bahia	Cod fish
Wasps	Johnson	Other fish
Hornets	**Trees**	Shrimp
Yellow jackets	Birch	Other shellfish
Fire ants	Beech	Peanuts
Weeds	Oak	Other legumes
Ragweed	Cedar	Wheat
Plantain	Olive	Soy
Mugwort	Palm	Eggs
Pigweed	Hickory	Milk
Lambs quarter	Poplar (cottonwood)	Tree nuts and seeds

Note: The theme running through this list is that all these are plant or animal compounds. There's nothing here to suggest that Aqua Velva or Xerox toner would likely enter the realm of acceptable immunotherapy any time soon.

"Good" Immunotherapy and "Bad"

The science of extracting allergens to create allergy shots has progressed tremendously in the many years since we began practice. Back then, a company in North Carolina purchased dust swept by a group of church-going women in the area to make the serum. Now we know that dust allergy is caused by a single protein in the fecal matter of dust mites, and it can be isolated and distilled to manufacture a much more effective (and hygienic) treatment.

With immunotherapy, as it is with all allergy-related medical care, a good history is the key to good treatment. The doctor's deductions should be supplemented by skin tests, which are both more accurate and less expensive than RAST tests.

Effective allergen-specific immunotherapy should also meet a number of criteria:

First, the allergic condition must be proven as responsive to allergy shots. The conditions currently recognized as falling into this category are allergic rhinitis, allergic conjunctivitis, asthma, hypersensitivity to fire ants and other hymenoptera, and drug allergy.

Second, the allergenic substances in the injectable vaccine should be specific to the allergy being treated and uncontaminated by extraneous allergens. That's not to say that several allergens can't be mixed into fewer shots by an allergist who knows what to consider in making combinations, because of course each child wants as few injections as possible. The allergist must consider the season, the dose of each allergen, and the compatibility of each allergen in the mixture.

Third, because shots increase in potency as immunity is built up, the allergens must also be strong enough at each level of treatment to provoke a maximal immune response.

Finally, the patient has to be dedicated. He has to stick to the whole course of treatment and not stop when he thinks he is all better. He also should avoid alternative forms of immunotherapy, claims for which may sound better than this long-haul pain in the neck, but are unproven. These are: *low-dose injections*, which aren't strong enough to build immunity; *oral treatments*, which are so damaged by the digestive system that there's little allergen left to provoke an immune response; *enzyme-potentiated therapy*; and, in the current state of science, *food allergy injections*.

Playing It Safe

Allergen immunotherapy, fast or slow, always involves injecting substances to which the patient is known to be allergic. Therefore, unwanted or even dangerous reactions are always possible. These range from itchy, localized swelling to systemic and even fatal anaphylaxis.

These complications can come from any number of factors: errors in dosage, active asthma, extreme hypersensitivity, use of beta-blockers, injections from a new vial that might be contaminated (although this rarely happens), mixtures that are too strong (which is more frequent), and injections during a season when allergies are at their peak.

Fortunately fatalities are extremely rare, not only because the practice of immunotherapy is very good but also because we take rescue precautions. We keep patients on hand for twenty to thirty minutes after giving a shot, and longer for patients who have had difficulty with the treatment. Epinephrine—adrenaline—is given for extreme reactions.

Future Shots

Current research holds the promise of much safer courses of immunotherapy. One promising avenue is changing the allergy material so that it provokes a good immune response but without being allergenic enough to provoke an allergic response. This is much like a classic vaccination.

Another exciting development, now in final stages of evaluation, is the second type of allergy shot we alluded to early in the chapter, and which we refer to elsewhere in the book. This is anti-IgE, in effect *an antibody to the allergic antibody*, which would be injected into the blood stream or beneath the skin and accomplish what would otherwise require a lengthy course of traditional allergy shots. If you block or neutralize the functioning of the allergic antibody IgE, allergies get better. Laboratory anti-IgE has shown in trials to effectively improve asthma and allergies, including peanut allergy, the most critical and stubborn food-allergic problem. It also helps remove IgE antibodies, accelerating the traditional immunotherapy process. Thus, high or maintenance levels of allergy vaccine may be administered much sooner than with conventional immunotherapy.

Antibodies At War

Yes, we now have antibodies against antibodies. You may recall that we said all classes of antibodies look like a lobster, its two claws reacting to antigens such as ragweed or bacteria. The tails of each class are different in that they set off a reaction unique to that class. Allergic IgE antibody tails are buried in the mast cell surface. When their claws attach to an allergen, they cause the mast cell to fire off histamine and other bad stuff.

The first commercial anti-IgE antibody, omalizumab, sold under the name Xolair, was created by genetic engineering, although when something costs $1,000 per month the word "commercial" must be used with a touch of irony.

Xolair acts like a laser-guided smart bomb, seizing allergic IgE antibodies from the blood by their tails. The tail of the IgE remains buried in the mast cell untouched.

At present, the cost of Xolair limits its use to mild-to-severe persistent asthmatics with elevated IgE who have undergone at least one course of steroids. Depending on the patient's weight and IgE level, Xolair is given every two to four weeks for an indefinite period. This reduces IgE levels by 50–90 percent and incidence of asthma by 50 percent, which is much faster than traditional allergy injections. By only lowering the allergic antibody, however, Xolair does not create protective antibodies. Traditional allergy injections do both over a

---

XOLAIR SAVES THE BRIDE

I was called to the emergency room to consult on a young woman with asthma. After the crisis was over, I noticed her ring finger was held in a way I have noticed is characteristic of newly engaged women as they get accustomed to displaying a shining rock.

I asked her if she knew what she is allergic to, and she replied, "I have been tested three times and each time I got a severe reaction to the tests. I would like to get better before the wedding."

I thought, since I can't do skin tests I'll try blood tests instead. Not only were the blood tests positive to certain allergens, but her total allergic antibody level was very high.

I said, "With your history and IgE level, regular injections might be too risky; I would like to try Xolair."

She said, "OK Doc, just make me better before the wedding." The she added, "I'm marrying a marine." Not as a threat, I believe.

With Xolair she was better in two months, and I was invited to a wedding at Camp Lejeune.
                                        — *Dr. Chiaramonte*

longer period of time. The anti-allergic response is thus slower but more complete.

In the crucible of the FDA approval process a choice must be made between limiting the claims for Xolair or continuing with extremely expensive research. Currently, claims are limited to patients with allergic antibody IgEs up to 700 units; for use with patients who exceed that level, a new and costly investment will be required to gain approval.

There are practical considerations in giving Xolair. Administering the medication requires more than two and a half hours. The doctor and patient must fight the insurance company for approval throughout the course of treatment, which may prevent the timely arrival of medication. Often when the patient shows improvement, the insurance uses this as a reason to withdraw approval and the patient returns to his former state. In anticipation that insurance coverage of Xolair will be withdrawn, we have started using traditional immunotherapy along with the Xolair in hopes of maintaining the dramatic improvement from the initial anti-IgE treatment.

So for the allergy patient, some things are getting better all the time, in theory anyway; the biggest problem of treatment is its cost.

Compliance, Compliance, Compliance

Compliance—sticking to a treatment routine—is a running theme in this book. The effectiveness of allergy treatment, like the management of any other chronic disease, rises and falls with the patient's adherence to a routine. Immunotherapy is no different than any other kind of regimen in this respect, which is a shame since it is the only therapy that offers relief from routine. That is, it changes the body in ways that make it easier to live a regular life—by eating more foods, taking part in more activities, and enjoying different environments without constantly worrying about allergies and taking medications.

There is no denying, however, that some people find the weekly or monthly routine of dropping around to the doctor for a shot intolerable.

We have done all we could: We have combined the sera for multiple allergies into a single shot. We have reduced the frequency from weekly to monthly, where possible. We prepare months of treatments in advance and provide them to patients' primary care physicians if it's more convenient to go to the GP or pediatrician than to come to our offices. Yet, even that is too much for some.

Under the Tongue

The latest wrinkle is called sublingual immunotherapy, which goes by the somewhat creepy acronym SLIT. Sublingual means "under the tongue." SLIT is used more often in Europe than it is in the U.S., which we suspect may be due in part to the fact that the acronym doesn't have the same connotations that it does here. Regardless, we still have a long regulatory road ahead before it gains the same level of use here as across the Atlantic. Efficacy for more than the current limited number of allergens will also have to be proven before we use it more widely.

The idea of sublingual immunotherapy is attractive, especially for pediatric allergists. We would have to give fewer of those painful shots. There's also the fact that it could be taken at home, which would save the health care system money.

There are two big drawbacks in the long run. First would be that we wouldn't be in a position to monitor bad reactions. And the second is that left to their own devices, many patients wouldn't follow

---

WORTH A TRY

With the increasing acceptance of SLIT therapy in this country and my perception of its convenience, I put five patients on this therapy. One patient was myself. The results were surprising:

1. One patient who accepted cockroach extract by subcutaneous injection, refused to take it orally. I wonder why.

2. Another patient complained of a burning sensation in his mouth on every ingestion of oral antigen.

3. The three remaining patients (including myself) found weekly subcutaneous immunotherapy to be more convenient than daily oral/sublingual immunotherapy.

My enthusiasm for SLIT has waned. The FDA and most insurance companies consider sublingual immunotherapy "investigational" as a technique of allergy immunotherapy. — *Dr. Chiaramonte*

---

their treatment, as we mention above. In the meantime, we have many decades of experience with subcutaneous injections. We know they work.

Still, while SLIT remains a work in progress, it is worth pursuing.

CHAPTER 10

Back to the Future?
Alternative Treatment for Allergies
And Asthma

INTEREST IN "ALTERNATIVE" MEDICAL TREATMENT—THAT IS, TREAT-
ment outside the mainstream of what is deemed effective by
medical boards and other authorities—has itself reached the
mainstream. There is now a government agency, part of the National
Institutes of Health, devoted to exploring alternative medicine, and
some of the most interesting science being done under grants from the
NIH at New York's Mount Sinai School of Medicine use traditional
Chinese herbal medicine to treat eczema, asthma, and food allergies.
More about that later.

We can understand the attraction of alternative treatment. It
seems to hold the promise of a cure or at least control of conditions
that range from the merely annoying to the life threatening without
the expense and discipline of advanced chemistry. The problem will
always be: Where does medicine end and quackery begin?

Suspicion of conventional medicine is understandable. After all,
part of the current rising incidence of allergies and asthma can be
attributed to "progress." That is, among other things, people who live
in modern, energy-efficient homes are more prone to allergy because
of that very energy efficiency; reduction of fresh air circulation to
keep homes cool in the summer and warm in the winter makes them
better breeding grounds for dust mites. Good modern engineering
thus unlocks long-dormant immune mechanisms in the genes. What
once saved people from parasites today makes their descendants
miserable.

Furthermore, as we have already indicated, much of what people
consider mainstream—the treatment they receive from their GPs and
pediatricians—gives mainstream medicine a bad name. "I'm sick, and
the doctor gives me medication that makes me feel sicker or affects

172

affects other parts of my body, and it costs too much money to boot."

Is there anything to alternative treatments? Yes and no. Yes to the extent that over many centuries, people around the world have lived with a genetic disposition to allergy and have tried many different remedies, some of which have worked. No to the extent that they should not be considered a substitute for modern treatment until they are proven effective. That is why the work at Mount Sinai is so intriguing; it is subject to all the necessary protocols.

As physicians, bound by the Hippocratic Oath, our responsibility is "first do no harm." It is one thing for people to drink green tea because they have read that there is something in it that will help with their allergic rhinitis—it may not be true, but it can't hurt. Former New York Yankees manager Joe Torre drank it constantly in the dugout during games, and probably still does in his current job with the Dodgers. (It is part of his post-cancer routine.) If nothing else, drinking hot drinks can loosen up the sinuses. But it is something else entirely when people rub primrose oil on eczema or let someone stick needles in their back to cure asthma instead of taking their maintenance doses of dry powder anti-inflammatory medicines.

Nothing would please us more than to find some shortcut to better health for our patients. We would be delighted to find some mechanism that would allow their bodies to heal themselves. But it probably won't happen soon. In the meantime, we must apply our medical knowledge and experience to alternative treatments just as we would anything that came from the laboratories of Glaxo or Merck.

Culture and Medicine

In New York, arguably the most ethnically diverse city in the world, we see an incredible range of folk wisdom in our offices.

For example, Puerto Ricans, Dominicans, and other Latinos distinguish between *caliente* (hot) medicines and *frio* (cold) medicines. Aspirin—the most widely used anti-inflammatory medicine in the world—is *caliente* because at some point people began using it during cold weather to treat the pain of arthritis. (The whole idea is that you treat a "cold" disease with a "hot" medicine and vice versa, and since arthritis comes when you are cold, aspirin must be a hot medicine.)

But because it is now a "hot" medicine, these Puerto Ricans do not consider it appropriate for treating the "heat" of fever, when in fact its anti-inflammatory properties make it effective for that, too. Yet, while avoiding aspirin may hinder treatment of the inflammation of fever, it can actually be a benefit for asthmatics. Some people experience asthma symptoms after taking aspirin or similar nonsteroidal anti-inflammatory drugs (NSAIDs) such as acetaminophen, ibuprofen, and naproxen, medications that alter the balance of mediators that control inflammation and bronchial constriction.

A 2002 study of asthma in a Dominican community published in the *Journal of Pediatric Psychology* (vol. 27, 4:385–392) dealt with just this topic. The mothers would use prescription medication for asthma attacks, and use them until the episode stopped, even if prescribed for longer.

To prevent asthma attacks, these mothers dressed their kids warmly: "[The majority of mothers] attributed the cause of their children's asthma attacks at school to teachers who permitted them to go outside in cold weather." To control asthma, the mothers preferred *zumos* (folk remedies) in place of standard therapies—concoctions made of things like whale oil, cod liver oil, honey, royal jelly, onion, garlic, almond oil, castor oil, oregano, lemon, and aloe vera juice.

While we have made great strides in treating previously insular communities in New York, the lessons of this study must be learned again and again, not just in ethnic enclaves, and not just among the disadvantaged. Namely, that the biggest barrier to effective compliance is inadequate communication. A mother put it very eloquently to the researchers: "The doctors don't take the time to explain things to me … When he was four, they told me that he had asthma, but I don't know because doctors never tell the truth. [Why not?] So one will not get worried … They don't tell you what the consequences might be so parents won't stop using the medicines, because if one knows then one would stop using them. They have a lot of patients so I know I can't ask many questions because they are busy."

If doctors, nurses, and social workers don't take the time to talk with patients and their parents, rich or poor, they will never take the new treatments to heart, and change their behavior in ways that will keep asthma under permanent control.

A TEACHER LEARNS A LESSON

When I was teaching asthma and allergy to young physicians, we found that most of our asthma patients came from a poor black area of Brooklyn. We enlisted the aid of a Jamaican asthma drug salesman to help us run a local asthma information program. On his advice we approached a church to host our teaching day, which they were only too glad to do. The minister was showing us the stained glass windows from the days of the church's former glory when I noticed some bullet holes from a drive-by shooting. I thought to myself: This is why it is so difficult to get these asthmatics to think of prevention; they have to think about staying alive day to day.

We wanted to get a "draw"—someone the people would come out to see. All the sports figures wanted too much money. The best we could do was a politician did tell his story of growing up with asthma. In this poor area, I learned how hard our treatments were to implement.

I had asked a black woman I once taught who was by now a certified allergist to talk to the people there. To my dismay she began by talking not about our new scientific treatments, but about folk treatments from Africa and the American South, how grand-mothers could replace doctors in a pinch, and how people would use cat's milk to treat asthma. She now had the attention of the people in a way I never could, and began to convince them to start with the scientific treatments. The distance from the folk remedies to the modern treatment was not as great as I thought, but it took the right messenger to lead them across the bridge.

I asked my Jamaican asthma drug salesman what he thought. He said, "Those treatments are from the South—we have our own treatments in Jamaica."
                                                              — *Dr Chiaramonte*

Compliance and the Search for Alternatives

Why people seek alternatives to the kind of medicine MDs practice depends in part on the patient's "belief system," which underpins the practice of medicine in every culture. After all, a tribal shaman or witchdoctor can be an effective healer, at least temporarily. Why? One part is because, as you will read, herbs and barks can contain real medicinal chemicals that are used in modern medicines. The other part is that they and their patients trust the treatment.

What does "belief" mean in medicine?

First, there's the confidence the doctor displays in administering a treatment. One-third of patients will get better on injections of saline if the doctor appears to have faith in it. It might have something to do with the fact that stress aggravates asthma—and when you take treatment with confidence that it will work, stress can be temporarily relieved. The doctor's belief or disbelief is contagious (forgive the pun). You may remember that the actor Robert Young, who played Marcus Welby, MD on TV, did commercials for medicine. How many people actually thought he was a real life doctor? When Ronald Reagan defeated Jimmy Carter for the presidency, was it because people thought he was smarter than Carter, who had, after all, been trained in nuclear physics? Probably not, but Reagan, with all his years in Hollywood and on television, certainly played the part of President better than Carter.

The other half of the equation, of course, is that the patient—or the patient's parent—must also believe. If a child has been treated ineffectively by GPs or non-allergist specialists, he will grow skeptical of doctors.

At least part of the problem, as we see it, is in what we refer to as compliance. Simply put, patients don't do what their doctors tell them to do. There's that phrase "used as directed." Lots of people don't and the medicine doesn't work. Dr. Sanders at Yale says that an important component of compliance is to explain the whys of treatments.

The authors of the article on Dominican mothers say, "Their cultural belief systems about health and illness are logically consistent and coherent to these mothers, they do not see themselves as being noncompliant or failing to provide adequate care ... Hence, it becomes our responsibility to acknowledge their folk beliefs about asthma and the home remedies they use in order to break the taboo about discussing differing belief systems about illness management."

With asthma medications, three things affect compliance. One is that people don't trust steroids even though, as we have said before, they are safe and the most effective medicines we have. Because they don't trust the medications, they don't use them as often as they should, and the lack of effectiveness becomes self-fulfilling.

Next is ease of use. Most people prefer to drive a car with an automatic transmission and not a manual, even if the manual gets better gas mileage. Likewise, the more complicated it is to administer a drug and the more regularly it has to be taken, the less likely a patient will be fully compliant. Drugs you can take once or twice a day can be left at home and used in the morning or the evening. But more often than that, they have to be carried around. They are easily lost, and of course, your child has to remember to take them. There may be difficulty in inhaling properly, and finally, with children, there's the all-important criterion: How does it taste?

Finally, for parents, there is the matter of cost. Most medicines are covered by insurance, but co-payments increase with nongenerics, and even with low co-payments the bill can add up if several prescriptions are involved. A newer, easy-to-use powder inhaler like Advair runs about $200 a month so insurance carriers prefer older, harder-to-take drugs.

All this adds up to an obstacle course that when taken together will sabotage effective treatment, and thus drive people towards cheaper, easier, and possibly crazier alternatives.

What Does the Literature Say About Alternatives?

The discussion that follows is mostly limited to studies we have read about in the literature. Let's face it: Our orientation in the kind of Western-style medicine that some patients find problematic doesn't give us much basis for first-hand experience with acupuncture or herbal tea. However, we do now and then see patients who have dabbled in these things, and sooner or later, they're back on pharmaceuticals under our care.

Asian cultures are particularly big on herbal treatments, as well as techniques like acupuncture, which are likely to be very appealing to patients and their families. Chinese, Japanese, Indian, and Korean variations have all been studied and there is evidence of effectiveness. But are they better than what we have to offer? The fact that many of these remedies were used for hundreds of years before the development of medical science as we know it is good enough for some people. But not for us. The fact is, while many herbs, teas, and barks may have medicinal qualities, they are medicinal because they contain chemicals that are just as potent as anything produced in a laboratory. People who extol "natural" remedies because they are natural are fooling themselves. Hemlock is natural, but, as Socrates found out, it is also fatal.

A look at the chemistry of many Asian asthma and allergy treatments, after you get past the exotic names, yields a familiar name—ephedra—the synthetic version of which, ephedrine, is an active ingredient in many over-the-counter preparations in U.S. drugstores. It is also the active ingredient in crystal meth, which is why meth "cookers" will go to great lengths to steal commercial preparations that contain ephedrine from drugstores.

The Chinese herbal remedy *ma huang* has been shown to pose significant central nervous system and cardiovascular risks because it contains ephedra, which is the same as ephedrine. It also has been linked to sudden death from ephedrine toxicity, nephrolithiasis, and acute hepatitis. Ephedra-derived weight-loss medicines made the headlines in the winter of 2003 because they were linked to the death of a minor league baseball pitcher at spring training with the Baltimore Orioles, as well as previous fatalities in other sports.

The *Kampo* formulations used for centuries by Japanese practitioners can result in fatal liver or kidney failure, and pneumonia and pneumonitis have been reported with the use of *Saiboku-to*.

The point of this discussion is not to endorse or condemn any treatment. Probably every ethnic group has some treatment of its own. As you will see, there are many methods that have some basis in reality. But we also recommend that you not use these treatments without recognizing their limitations, and without consultation with a qualified allergist.

Warning: Look Out for Quacks

Here are some things to look out for if you are tempted by alternative treatment:

• **Quick or simple cures** One size doesn't fit all, and regardless, if something seems too good to be true, it probably is, as we learned from the subprime mortgage market.

• **Diets** Food is part of the answer in some cases, but it's not the whole story.

• **Money** Will a reputable insurance company pay for part or all of the treatment? While we are no great admirers of insurance companies and health maintenance organizations, better known as HMOs, they are often a fairly reliable indicator of what has achieved recognition through scientific trial and what has not. Beware of anything

---

BUYER BEWARE

One website espousing a particular therapy says:
"[B]ronchitis, pneumonia, and asthma ... chest muscle pains, poor circulation, rapid heartbeats, heart irregularities ... acute abdominal pains, acute appendicitis, bloating, constipation, diarrhea and ulcers ... kidney and bladder infections, prostate troubles, pre-menstrual syndromes and post menstrual disorders, impotency, infertility ... unexplained pains anywhere in the body, various types of headaches, backaches, arthritis, restless leg syndrome, brain symptoms like brain fog, depression, anger, attention-deficit disorders, hyperactivity, learning disorders, skin problems like eczema, boils, slow healing wounds, environmental re8actions like multiple chemical sensitivity, allergy to pollens, perfumes, animal dander, carpets, building materials, etc... *just about any health condition could be merely a symptom of underlying allergies.* [Italics added.]

"And where do allergies come from?:

"When contact is made with an allergen, it causes blockages in the energy pathways called meridians, or we can say, it disrupts the normal flow of energy through the body's electrical circuits. This energy blockage causes interference in communication between the brain and body via the nervous system.

"And how are allergies treated [using the doctor's method]?:

"Allergens are cleared (treated) one at a time with [the doctor's proprietary] technique, and best results are obtained if allergens are cleared in a specific sequence. Normally only one item is treated on a given day. The substance must then be completely avoided for 25 hours following the treatment. In most cases, that's all it takes ... one session to eliminate an allergy. Individuals who are highly sensitive may sometimes require additional combination clearings."

---

that's either too cheap or too expensive. Some quacks, like narcotics dealers, make money by dispensing their snake oil in small doses over a long period of time. Others prefer to charge exorbitant fees in advance.

• **Books for sale** We recognize that this is a strange criterion, considering the circumstances. But ours is not the kind of book we are talking about. We are talking about those that make it all too simple, by authors whose credentials are in fields other than medicine, and which are promoted on talk shows with a testimonial or two from those who have miraculously been cured.

• **Diet supplements** The generic name for this is snake oil. Even when the supplement involves one of the vitamins or minerals discussed here, look skeptically at broad claims.

Emotion and Asthma

The most important alternatives deal with emotional health, and in fact, emotional stress has long been linked to asthma. Traditional Chinese medicine recognizes a connection between the lungs and grief, a linkage borne out by modern psychology. Recent studies have found greater anxiety and depression among asthma patients than other people, including those who suffer from a number of other chronic diseases.

With apologies to people with food allergies, there's a chicken-or-egg element to this discussion. Namely, do asthma patients have anxiety and depression because of their asthma, or do anxiety and depression predispose them to asthma symptoms? It may be a combination.

Undoubtedly, shortness of breath and heavy wheezing can be pretty anxiety producing. Conversely, intense emotions can bring also precipitate asthma symptoms. Respiratory resistance, airway reactivity, shortness of breath, and decreased peak expiratory flow rate have all been shown to occur after an emotional challenge.

Biofeedback

We have seen the efficacy of biofeedback training in our practice, and in fact have published research on the subject. Relaxation and beneficial slow, deep, diaphragmatic breathing from biofeedback decrease symptom severity, decrease medication usage, decrease emergency room visits, and increase lung function values. Transcendental Meditation training produces similar results.

In a study we published fifteen years ago, we were able to block the "asthma inducing" medication, methacholine, after teaching patients with asthma a method of biofeedback.

Yoga Breathing

Yoga, which emphasizes breathing techniques, has also been shown to help asthma patients. Hundreds of patients who were taught yoga demonstrated significant improvement in asthma symptoms, medication usage, peak flow rate, and exercise tolerance. Transcendental Meditation and other forms of meditation produce similar results.

Nutrients and Asthma

Because of the biochemistry involved in asthma and allergy, there's logic in a link between nutrients and these conditions. We would caution, however, that you take any extravagant promises about nutrition-based treatments with more than just the proverbial grain of salt. Certain nutrients are harmless when taken in large quantities. (Americans are said to have the world's most expensive urine because they take more water-soluble vitamins than they need, which just pass through them.) Some vitamins and other nutrients, on the other hand, can hurt you. All the nutrients we discuss here have peer-reviewed research or other respectable support behind them.

Vitamin D

Unlike many other vitamins, vitamin D gets plenty of respect. The body naturally manufactures its own D when our skin is exposed to sunshine. Cow's milk generally has vitamin D added. Between those two sources, children have traditionally gotten all they need. However, today they are likely to drink less milk and get less sunshine in routine play. Sunscreens, which are routinely used at the beach, also interfere with vitamin D synthesis. Adults get commensurately less of each, and moderate supplementation is recommended for many reasons, including bone health. Now add asthma to the list.

One of the most respected asthma research and treatment facilities in the world, National Jewish Hospital in Denver, found that vitamin supplementation may improve response to inhaled steroids. Rand Sutherland, MD, MPH, chief of the pulmonary division at National Jewish, says, "Our findings suggest that vitamin D levels influence a number of important features of asthma, including lung function, bronchospasm, and therapeutic response to steroids."

Vitamin C

There is reason to believe "oxygen radicals" play a part in the pathophysiology of bronchial asthma. Inflammatory cells generate and release reactive oxygen species—loose oxygen atoms that can cause damage to the lungs and other body parts—that are absorbed by vitamin C. Inflammatory cells from asthma patients produce more reactive oxygen species than those of nonasthmatics. The lung lining fluid of asthmatics shows significantly lower levels of vitamin C and vitamin E than normal, even though plasma levels were normal.

Children with asthma were found to have significantly decreased serum levels of vitamin E, beta-carotene, and vitamin C even when they had no symptoms, and higher levels of lipid peroxidation products during attacks. Using antioxidant nutrients might be helpful in combating the increased oxidant levels in asthmatics.

Epidemiological studies on respiratory function note a beneficial overall effect on respiratory function from taking vitamin C. Yet the effect of vitamin C on asthma remains controversial, because studies have yielded contradictory results.

Allergy patients occasionally complain of increased sensitivity to mosquito bites, which makes sense because they are allergic to proteins in the mosquito venom. I was told by one patient twenty years ago that vitamin B$_6$ taken during the summer "warded off" mosquitoes. Having suggested its use with the warning that it might not work, I observed that some, but not all, found it very helpful. *Caveat emptor.* If you are bitten, oral and topical antihistamines can help

— *Dr. Ehrlich*

Vitamin B$_6$

Pyridoxal 5'-phosphate (PLP), the active form of vitamin B$_6$ in the body, is involved in many biochemical processes, and has been found in lower concentrations in asthma patients. However, studies of the therapeutic efficacy of B$_6$ supplementation have produced mixed results. One showed that treating asthmatic adults with pyridoxine (50 mg twice daily) reduced asthma exacerbation and wheezing episodes. A study of children showed that B$_6$ supplementation (100 mg pyridoxine hydrochloride twice daily) resulted in fewer bronchoconstrictive attacks; less wheezing, coughing, and chest tightness; and lower usage of bronchodilators and steroid medications. However, a double-blind trial of B$_6$ (300 mg per day pyridoxine hydrochloride) in steroid-dependent asthma patients showed no change in lung function.

Asthma patients treated with the bronchodilator theophylline have lower blood levels of PLP, though it is not used as often as it once was. Patients using this drug should be monitored for vitamin B$_6$ levels and supplements should be given if warranted.

Vitamin B$_{12}$

It has been reported that children with asthma may be deficient in B$_{12}$. Although there is no peer-reviewed literature to corroborate such a statement, some think that B$_{12}$ supplementation will be helpful to some children, particularly if they are sulfite-sensitive.

Magnesium

Magnesium plays a part in over 300 biochemical processes in the body. It works with calcium to regulate contraction and relaxation of smooth muscle, which makes it important to breathing. Calcium helps the muscles contract, while magnesium helps them relax. Asthmatics commonly have low levels of magnesium, and in more severe cases they are lower still. Without the relaxation promoted by magnesium, the calcium keeps muscles in an over-contracted state.

Intravenous magnesium sulfate is a vital component of emergency asthma treatment in many hospitals. Often, symptoms are relieved soon after infusion begins, which can decrease the need for intubation.

While the results of studies using magnesium sulfate are inconsistent, asthmatics do tend to have lower intracellular magnesium levels, and supplementation to correct those levels seems warranted.

Zinc

Zinc deficiency by itself has not been linked to asthma symptoms, but asthma patients have been shown to have lower plasma zinc than healthy subjects. Serum and hair zinc have been found to be significantly lower in individuals with asthma and atopic dermatitis.

Even without definitive research on long-term zinc use for asthmatics, such supplementation appears to be warranted to avoid potential exacerbation of asthma symptoms.

Selenium

Glutathione peroxidase (GSH-Px) is an enzyme that contains selenium that uses glutathione to help metabolize hydrogen peroxide, thus protecting against oxidative damage. Individuals with asthma tend to have higher oxidative activity, lower levels of selenium, and diminished glutathione peroxidase activity.

There's been just one study on the effects of selenium supplementation on the increased pulmonary oxidative burden in asthmatics, which showed increases in serum and platelet selenium and GSH-Px activity. Improvements in subjective symptomatology were also observed. However, objective measurements of lung function showed no change.

Omega-3 Fatty Acids

Some of the most important mediators of allergic activity, notably prostaglandins and leukotrienes, are intermediate and end products of fatty acid metabolism. Research into the effects of leukotrienes has spurred the development of new drugs to block their activity, and appear to be of benefit in some asthma patients, particularly those with more severe disease.

When cold-water fatty fish containing relatively large amounts of the omega-3 fatty acids eicosapentaenoic acid (EPA) and docosahexaenoic acid (DHA) are eaten, or when their oil is taken as a supplement, EPA and DHA displace arachidonic acid from cell membranes. These cells subsequently release relatively higher concentrations of fish-derived oils. The end products are mediators that are less inflammatory than normal. This shift toward less inflammatory mediators would lead us to expect to see less inflammatory activity in the lungs, and a subsequent improvement in asthma symptoms. Epidemiological studies do show that the more fish we eat, the less risk of asthma. However, the clinical data is equivocal when it comes to taking omega-3 fatty acid supplements, with studies showing both positive and negative results.

Botanicals and Asthma

Arguments for saving the rain forest include the possibility that undiscovered species of plants will some day cure everything from the common cold to cancer. Herbalists and naturopaths use a number of botanicals to relieve symptoms of asthma—expectorants such as lobelia, sanguinaria, and grindelia, for example—although we aren't aware of any that have undergone the kind of trial that would qualify it for basic clinical treatment in our practice. Such a plant derivative would have to show effectiveness against excess histamine release, leukotriene synthesis, and unbalanced immune activity. However, the following botanicals and derivatives seem to have some efficacy in treating asthma:

Tylophora asthmatica

An Indian plant called *Tylophora asthmatica* (also known as *Tylophora indica* or Indian ipecac) has undergone clinical scrutiny and shown success in treating asthma. The leaves are used in Indian medicine—also known as Ayurvedic medicine—for treating asthma, bronchitis, and arthritis. It can have an irritant effect on the gastrointestinal mucosa and in large doses, as every parent should know, will act as an emetic. In smaller doses, however, it acts as an expectorant and anti-inflammatory, and may provide benefit in asthma cases.

Alkaloids from this plant called tylophorine and tylophorinine are believed to account for the plant's efficacy. A rat study of tylophorine showed that it inhibited systemic anaphylaxis, adjuvant-induced arthritis, and mast-cell degranulation.

Ingestion of *Tylophora* leaf in asthma patients resulted in improvements in asthma symptoms at night, as well as significant improvements in lung function indices compared to placebo in a double-blind, crossover study.

Boswellia serrata

The gum resin of *Boswellia serrata*—known popularly as frankin-cense—has been used in Ayurvedic medicine for centuries, and is also known as Salai guggul. Components of *Boswellia* called boswellic acids have been found to specifically inhibit 5-lipoxygenase, an enzyme that helps produce leukotrienes, which contribute to inflammation. In animal studies, *Boswellia* not only inhibited production, but also prevented the migration of leukocytes to inflammatory sites. This inhibitory effect might make it a useful component of therapy, and clinical trials have been encouraging.

Plant Sterols and Sterolins

One of the basic biochemical dysfunctions in allergy is the increase of the immunoglobulin IgE and specific T-cell activity. Overactive Th2 cells increase IgE antibody formation, chemotaxis of neutrophils, and eosinophilia, leading to an improper immune and inflammatory response.

A hopeful line of research treatment lies with plant sterols and sterolins (sterol glycosides). A blend of these (in a ratio of 100:1) has been shown to increase Th1 activity while dampening Th2 in animals and humans with chronic viral infections, tuberculosis and HIV. Clinical studies of this compound are ongoing for treatment of the immune system–related diseases rheumatoid arthritis, HIV, hepatitis C, human papilloma virus, and asthma/allergic rhinitis. Research-based evidence is currently lacking for asthma.

Hands-On Treatments

Massage

Regular massage therapy can benefit asthma patients by relaxing the musculature and reducing anxiety. A study of children with asthma who received massage daily for thirty days demonstrated increased peak airflow and FEV_1 during the course of the study.

Chiropractic/Osteopathic Manipulation

This is a problematic area for us as physicians. We wonder whether benefits shown after these practitioners perform spinal adjustments on asthma patients are because of reduced anxiety, similar to the improvements of massage, or because of the validity of their "medical" theory. We have a tough time with the chiropractic theory that attributes all disease to misalignment of the vertebrae, which can be treated by twisting a patient's neck. While spinal adjustments certainly can help an individual breathe better when there's a structural and neurological problem that makes breathing more difficult, asthma and allergy have biochemical bases that will not respond to a glorified back rub.

Acupuncture

A number of studies have been conducted on the effect of acupuncture on asthma symptoms, but unfortunately many suffer from methodology and/or data-reporting shortcomings, making it difficult to draw accurate conclusions. Another obstacle to good scientific study is the use of "sham" acupuncture, or placebo acupuncture, performed by non-acupuncturists. When real acupuncture is practiced, some research indicates that it can be beneficial. However, people have died because their asthma remained untreated except for acupuncture, while others have died of wounds because their "puncture" wasn't "acu" enough. Before we can be convinced of its efficacy in our practice, and where asthma is serious, never buy the promises of acupuncturists that your child doesn't need his medications.

Dr. Xiu Min Li and Chinese Medicine

As we said earlier, some of the most intriguing research in allergy science is being done at the Mount Sinai School of Medicine, directed by Beijing-born Dr. Xiu Min Li, Professor of Pediatrics in the Division of Pediatric Allergy and Immunology. We know Mount Sinai's allergy division: It is headed by our colleague Hugh Sampson, and Hugh knows talent when he sees it.

Dr. Li's work is grounded in traditional Chinese medicine. She collects ideas for the teas, ointments, and dietary supplements made from roots, herbs, and flowers from her collection of rare texts. These preparations have names like *Mai Men Dong Tang* and *Ding Chuan Tang*.

We have heard Dr. Li present her data, and she has published in the *Journal of Allergy and Clinical Immunology*, one of the premier publications in our field. While her chemistry is based on botanical alternatives to test-tube pharmaceuticals, the clinical practice in her clinic is subject to lengthy and exacting protocols, similar to those use for drugs made by Big Pharma, including measurement of IgE levels, and regular monitoring of patient health.

Pediatric patients for her practice typically arrive with eczema so bad and so resistant to conventional treatment that both parents and child are desperate. Many also have asthma and food allergies including peanut and shellfish allergy. Results for her work with all three categories are promising.

While we are very impressed by Dr. Li's work, it is no magic wand. Years of clinical trials lie ahead: One trial is in Phase Two, and another, just completed, was an extended Phase One (don't ask us to explain), involving patients aged 12 to 45. For asthma patients in particular, corticosteroid use remains the best means for controlling inflammation, and so cannot be stopped abruptly for any alternative treatment. Such treatment has to be done in tandem until patients are solidly symptom-free before they can be taken off steroids. Because there is no current treatment for food allergies except experimental immunotherapy and watching the diet, such a concurrent regimen isn't required, although avoiding anaphylaxis is still imperative. Likewise, eczema treatment isn't subject to the same kind of precise management as asthma, and so alternative treatment can also commence right away.

Before treatment, all patients have to undergo a battery of tests to assess organ function and general health. Although judging by thousands of years of use, herbal therapies are generally safe—the exceptions having been noted earlier in this chapter—Dr. Li's protocols further ensure safety and tolerability. While Dr. Li began to help patients with multiple allergic conditions at her clinic using traditional Chinese medicine under the category of dietary supplementation, this service is limited by standards of mainstream medical practice; i.e., once foods become drugs, they are regulated differently. Her work with a team of doctors and researchers at Mount Sinai Hospital and other medical centers has as its goal the development of prescription drugs (under the FDA botanical drug regulations) for treating allergies, so that physicians will have additional options to help their patients in the near future. Dr. Li is unique. She was trained in China and did pediatrics at Stanford and allergy and immunology at Johns Hopkins. She can read the basic texts in the original. Doctors like her will never roll off an assembly line. If she does succeed, the road to alternative treatments may be shorter than we once thought it would be, and it doesn't have to run past the traditional pharmacy or the health food store.

CHAPTER 11

Stages of an Allergic Life

POP QUIZ

1. If your little girl rubs the tip of her nose with her index finger and then with the palm of the hand upward towards her forehead, it means:

A. She is coming down with a cold.

B. She has disobeyed mommy and put beans in her nose.

C. She is performing what allergists call an "allergic salute."

2. If your 5-year-old boy has no history of respiratory problems but starts scratching his nose persistently in the evening before bed, it means:

A. He is thinking deeply.

B. He is working up to picking it after he goes to bed when no one is watching.

C. He should be tested for sensitivity to milk, cats, dust mites, molds, trees, ragweed, and grass.

3. If your 4-year-old son has recurring bronchiolitis and develops dark circles around his eyes, it means:

A. Congestion has made him irritable and he has gotten into a fight.

B. His school difficulties are causing him to lose sleep.

C. He has allergies.

4. Your 2-month-old son, born in July, starts getting red, rosy cheeks and his skin starts to itch at the height of ragweed season in September. He is probably:

A. Allergic to pollen.

B. Allergic to house dust mites.

C. Reacting to changes in the weather.

5. Your 3-year-old daughter starts getting congested at the end of ragweed season in the fall. She is probably:

A. Allergic to pollen.
B. Allergic to house dust mites.
C. Reacting to changes in the weather.

Answers:

1. C—Allergic salute. This is a specific behavior that all trained allergists recognize, but that might look like nothing out of the ordinary to a parent or pediatrician.

2. C—While your child is undoubtedly a deep thinker, these symptoms are typical of a few common sensitivities.

3. C—Congestion may be a symptom of many childhood conditions, but the dark circles are a tip-off: They are caused by chronic nasal congestion.

4. B—Allergic to house dust mites. How can we be so sure? Because he is encountering ragweed pollen for the first time at the age of 2 months, and thus has not been sensitized to it. His current problems are due to the household dust that he has been breathing for the past two months, unless there's a dog or cat in the house, in which case it might be them.

5. A—The flipside of the previous problem.

THE REASON FOR ASKING THESE QUESTIONS IS TO DEMONSTRATE that allergists are trained to look for certain symptoms that are not obvious to parents or even to pediatricians or general practitioners. Openly rubbing the nose is a part of childhood. Frequent minor infections are a fact of life for schoolchildren. Because such symptoms are common and seemingly minor, they are often overlooked or treated in the wrong ways—either as infections when they are allergy-related, or as allergy-related when they are not. Sometimes people think that they have suddenly become allergic as adults. This is probably not the case: Allergic symptoms begin at a very early age but they may not be recognized or treated as such, and the problem was worse years ago when today's parents were children.

We hope in this chapter to help you refocus your perception of your child's life—and your own—through the filter of allergy so that you have a better idea of how your family can adjust to the facts with minimal disruption.

Sherlock Holmes Again

All good doctors have a bit of Sherlock Holmes in them. Certain clues narrow the range of possibilities. Family practice and pediatrics are built around immediate problems, some very serious and some not. Ear infections. Sore throats. Stuffed noses. These may be routine and easily treated, but obviously, they can also be quite dangerous if wrongly diagnosed. The job of family doctors is to make sure that a garden-variety sore throat isn't strep. They must distinguish between the 90 percent of sore throats that will go away by themselves and the ones that must be treated with expensive antibiotics. They aren't trained to recognize obscure allergic symptoms.

Most allergies aren't life-threatening, although food and insect allergies and asthma can be. But they do take a toll on the quality of life—particularly heartbreaking in a child. How can a kid play ball when grass reduces him or her to sneezing, itching, and wheezing? Frequent absences from school can set the child back academically and socially.

By portraying Helen Hunt's son as a kid who was missing out on life, the Academy Award–winning movie *As Good As It Gets* gave a tremendous boost to the cause of publicizing the plight of childhood allergy sufferers. Because his mother had no health insurance, the poor boy was on a roller coaster of curtailed activity and emergency room visits. Sadly, this is all too common. It shouldn't be that way.

The long-term consequences can be significant, too. We once had one of the New York Yankees as a patient. He was allergic to grass and never made it past the level of a competent journeyman infielder. We can't say that if he had had better treatment at an early age he would have reached the Hall of Fame, but we can say that the sleeves of his uniforms would have been cleaner.

The field of allergy is more deductive than most. It takes time to learn what to look for, and it takes time with patients to learn family histories that might indicate allergies are present. Finally, it takes time to test for specific sensitivities once the likelihood of allergy is diagnosed. A GP or pediatrician doesn't have the kind of time it takes to learn these things or to act on them. The most time a general practitioner will ever take with a patient is during an initial physical, and then the family medical history has to include far more than allergic possibilities. When they do establish that some kind of allergic treatment is warranted, the economics of medicine today often dictate that the "gatekeeper" physician will try to provide treatment. However, the results of fee-for-service treatments, based on "doing rather than thinking" (in Dr. Sanders's words), are often scattershot and time-consuming and wrong. Physicians who are otherwise perfectly bright and competent make mistakes. They end up looking like Dr. Watson instead of Sherlock Holmes.

BRACE YOURSELF

Sometimes allergies turn up when you least expect them, unless you're an allergist. Take the case of 12-year-old Tommy. He had been a snorer for years, but no one thought much of it except the people within earshot when he was asleep, which did not include his pediatrician, naturally. However, the pediatrician did notice at a routine camp checkup that Tommy was developing an overbite and referred him to an orthodontist. The dentist applied braces with frequent return visits for tightening. Progress was slow. A snorer by night, it turns out that Tommy was a mouth breather by day. And because lip and tongue pressure against the upper palate are needed to help braces form a good dental arch, the orthodontist began exhorting Tommy to breathe through his nose. Tommy just couldn't do it because his nose was stuffed up. After discussion with the pediatrician, the dentist agreed that a visit to an allergist might help. An allergic treatment program for Tommy resulted in clearer nasal passages and much faster progress in correcting his overbite. — *Dr. Chiaramonte*

The Clock Starts Ticking Before Birth

The earliest indicators of allergy begin before a child is born. In fact, they begin before conception. One allergic parent creates a high probability of passing on susceptibility. With two, it's very high. Genetic research is only confirming what we have long observed, although it is revealing information that may some day lead to very precise therapy.

If life, broadly speaking, is unfair, a tendency to allergy makes it doubly unfair because the fuse may be lit unwittingly during pregnancy by the mother's eating habits. Eggs and dairy products, which are particularly nutritious and long recommended for prenatal diet, can sensitize the gestating child to certain allergens, precipitating some of the earliest allergic symptoms as little as a month after birth.

Poor sleeping, runny nose, dry skin—these are among the precursors to allergies that will escalate over the years. Moreover, they are so common that many times they will not even lead to a trip to the doctor. Instead, parents will live with the symptoms or treat them either with over-the-counter medications like Benadryl that may have sedating effects (which can't help his performance in school), or with folk remedies, but the child may be more sensitive than they can cope with. The result is misery for child and sympathetic suffering—frequently compounded by guilt—for the parents.

Fortunately, most GPs and pediatricians do now recognize the allergenic potential of infant diet. For example, while breast-feeding has had resurgence in the past thirty years, it doesn't necessarily protect the baby from allergies. A colicky baby may have sensitivity to something in the mother's diet—usually cow's milk or eggs. And while you wouldn't feed a baby a bottle of cow's milk in the first months of life, the major infant formulas are derived from cow's milk and can precipitate allergic symptoms. So an informed physician might move the baby rapidly to soy milk or other non-allergenic preparations, although in time the baby can become allergic to soy milk formula as well. However, here, as in all aspects of the allergy dilemma, the specialist will likely take a much more up-to-date, focused approach than the GP or pediatrician would be equipped for.

Furthermore, as we have said elsewhere in the book, the suspicion of food allergy, or even proven sensitivity to certain foods, can lead to the withholding of multiple foods to the point that the child becomes malnourished.

Anti-Allergic Prenatal Care

We can't choose our genes any more than we can choose our relatives, but we can take steps to minimize allergic symptoms as part of prenatal care. There are steps that couples with a family history of allergy can take prior to birth to minimize the symptoms that their child will experience:

• Test levels of IgE in umbilical cord blood; along with family history, this is a good predictor of future allergy.

• During last trimester of pregnancy (and during breast-feeding), mother should avoid high-allergy foods.

• Avoid exposure to dust mites by removing rugs in bedroom and covering mattresses.

• Keep no allergenic pets in home.

• Dad, get used to not smoking in front of child or quit altogether. (Mom should already have stopped.)

Clockwork Allergies

Allergies appear on a very predictable schedule, based on the range of allergens a child is routinely exposed to during successive stages of development. For example, colic appears in the first month of life based on exposure to proteins in the mother's diet during pregnancy.

The calendar is a key element in the allergist's medical diagnosis bag. As we point out in the pop quiz that opens this chapter, a July-born baby will show symptoms of congestion during the ragweed season not because of normal autumn pollens, but because of dust in the home or possibly a family pet. Same congestion, different cause, and consequently, different treatment.

ALLERGIC RESPONSE—THE SECOND TIME AROUND

An allergic response cannot take place upon first exposure to an allergen; sometimes that fact provides some very poignant glimpses into people's lives. For example, we once had a teenage patient from an observant Jewish family. His GP had ordered a standard battery of RAST tests and when son and father arrived to hear the results, I was chagrined to find a reaction to shrimp and lobster. These delicacies are not allowed under dietary laws observed by both devout Jews and Muslims, who are restricted to eating only *kosher* or *halal* foods, respectively. Ergo, it could only be that the son had tasted forbidden fruit of the sea.

In reviewing the results with them, my body language made the father suspicious and he asked to look at the printout himself. He said, "Doctor, it is my understanding that you only become allergic to things after you have already been exposed to them." I nodded. He turned to his son and spoke to him firmly but kindly in Yiddish. I couldn't contain my curiosity and asked him to tell me what he had said. He answered, "How did it taste?"

— *Dr. Ehrlich*

The reason it can't be ragweed is that ragweed is new that first autumn of life. Allergies only appear the second time around—when there are antibodies to the offending substance present to produce the response. As we say in our field, the system has to have "seen" the allergen. For the same reason, it's very likely that a year later the response will be to pollen. The child has been sensitized.

Allergy Timeline

As we said earlier, parental allergies are the best predictor of what's to come, although there are many variations. In general though, the timeline is pretty standard.

First weeks

• Colic. Indicative of allergy to components of formula, such as milk, eggs, and soy.

Up to 2 years of age

• Atopic dermatitis, eczema.
• Red, rosy cheeks, or "healthy baby" look. Progresses at a few years of age to dry, itchy skin and lichenification in the front of elbow (the *antecubital* area) and behind the knee (the *popliteal*).
• Recurring bronchiolitis (two or more episodes). Should prompt examination of family history, total IgE levels for age, and other signs of allergy.
• Food allergy. Immature digestive system absorbs whole proteins instead of breaking them down into useful components.

2 to 3 years of age

• Nasal symptoms with dark rings.
• Frequent ear infections (aerotitis, serositis). Until age 5 or 6.
• Asthma. Generally appears after age 2 and before age 10.

After 5 years of age

• Seasonal allergies. Become important after several pollen seasons and continual exposure to household allergens such as dust mites, molds, and cockroaches.

Telling Gestures

Allergic symptoms don't appear on cue in our offices any more than a car stalls in front of a mechanic, so we often need to assess our patients' allergies in the absence of immediate symptoms. One of the methods we use is to question patients and their parents about certain behaviors that indicate underlying allergy. We already described the "allergic salute," a very specific involuntary sequence of movements that indicates nasal allergies. There are others. For example, a clenched fist in the middle of the chest may look like someone having a heart attack, but when the patient is a child it probably means something else—tightening due to asthma.

We hope that by the time you finish reading this book, you will be a better observer of your child's allergic symptoms: not just overt ones like sneezing, but things like sleeping habits, moods, and so forth. This will make you a better guide for your child's pediatrician and allergist alike. A parent's concerned, loving observation is the front-line defense against allergy.

School Days

Pediatric allergists can plot their work year according to the school calendar. Right after school begins, when kindergartners and first graders pull out their mats and rugs at quiet time, we see a spate of dust-induced asthma and rhinitis. Guinea pigs and white mice are a soothing and educational addition to elementary classrooms, but they are also full of allergens.

When leaves start falling, mold spores begin to increase both indoors and out. At this time of year, air-temperature inversions—warm air on top of cold—occur both inside and out. This decreases the vertical mixing of air, and contaminants build up as a result.

The start of heating season is always busy in our offices. This is when custodians fire up the furnaces and all that dust and mouse droppings are swept from the heating ducts into the classroom.

On top of these seasonal events, schools remain an allergen super-market: Chalk, pollens, pesticides, laboratory chemicals, sanitation supplies, perfumes, rodents, and cockroaches all make schools a 7- to 10-hour-a-day, year-round threat.

According to the Environmental Protection Agency (EPA), nearly one in thirteen school-aged children has asthma, and the incidence of children with asthma is rising more rapidly in preschool-aged children than in any other age group. How does this affect their performance in school? Asthma accounts for over 10 million missed school days per year, making it the leading cause of school absenteeism from chronic illness. The nights of interrupted sleep, limitations on activity, and disruption of routines take a toll on concentration in class, homework quality, and general quality of life.

Some schools have made conscientious attempts to reduce exposure to allergens in schools, although there's still a great deal more to do. But even with considerate administrators and teachers, schools remain a roulette wheel as a 6-year-old patient of ours found out:

Scott, a first grader at a private school, is seriously allergic to peanuts. His mother informed the school. His teacher then went to the extent of telling the other children not to bring peanut butter for lunch, and the school nurse informed other parents, who were mostly happy to comply even though it complicated the job of making lunch. Scott, who was small and subject to teasing anyway, was now needled even more by his schoolmates. But one boy went further, smuggling peanut butter into the school, holding Scott down and forcing the stuff into his mouth. He almost died. The assailant was expelled.

Fortunately, such malicious acts are rare. But as with most things, it's not the extraordinary that represents the biggest threat, it's the ordinary. Still, we are against outright bans on peanuts because they are unenforceable in the long run. Kids make mistakes, or they cheat. The New York City Department of Education, which has more than 1,000 schools, will not institute a system-wide ban. We did, however, hear about a private school that, after a large donation from a grandparent, did ban them. Instead, we suggest that families take precautions on their own, and enlist key school personnel in the effort.

An Informed Child Is a Safe Child

The first line of defense, of course, is your own child. Make sure she knows her allergy and asthma triggers, symptoms, and treatment plan—and when to ask for help. With your physician, develop a written management plan for school and request that he get in touch with the principal and other health officials. It is unfortunate but often true that involving a physician will give your concerns more authority than you would have on your own. You should insist on meeting with your child's teacher, school health care staff, and food-service workers to review the plan and ensure everyone understands how to meet your child's needs.

If possible, reach out to the parents of other children in similar situations. Additional voices will not only reduce the sense of exceptionalism you and your child feel, it will make dramatic, systemic change more urgent—not a small problem in days of tight school budgets.

CHECKLIST FOR START OF SCHOOL YEAR

• Find out who staffs the health clinic. Do they know how to administer a metered-dose inhaler or nebulizer treatment for your child?

• Find out if school policy allows students to carry medication. If your child is old enough, make sure she knows how to use her medications.

• If students aren't permitted to carry medication, make sure the school staff knows where the medication is stored and how to administer it properly.

• Let the school know how to reach you during the day in case of an emergency.

• Tour your child's classroom before school starts to identify potential allergy and asthma triggers. Offer suggestions to protect your child's health.

• If your child has exercise-induced asthma, make sure coaches and physical education teachers know the warning signs and how to handle an emergency.

• When a child is itchy or can't breathe, it's hard to concentrate; both over-the-counter and prescription medicines can make them moody and impact their ability to learn. Work with your child's teacher to develop ways to help your child focus.

• Finally, keep lines of communication with the school open throughout the year. Review your management plan periodically and make sure everyone is comfortable with the strategies in place.

— *The MA Newsletter, August 2002*

Collective activity and information exchange are the crux of the work of organizations like Allergy & Asthma Network Mothers of Asthmatics (AANMA), which has been the clearinghouse for much useful information and tales of scientifically sound, grassroots efforts to make constructive change. Indeed, its newsletter, *The MA Report*, is a shortcut to help in changing your child's school for the better. AANMA may be contacted at 800-878-4403 or www.aanma.org.

Cleaner Air in School

How big a problem is the air in schools? In addition to the allergens that are prevalent in every school—what is a school without chalk after all?—most are poorly ventilated. Schools from the '70s were built to have low energy loss—an admirable goal itself. However, a certain amount of air circulation is required for people in a building, and a percentage of this should be fresh air from outside; some of these building went overboard trying to conserve energy and thus do not meet these standards. A February 1995 study of radon in schools by the Government Accountability Office (then known as the General Accounting Office) found that over half of those surveyed had poor ventilation, which traps allergens.

If there is any dampness in a building like this, a toxic mold called *Stachybotrys chartium* may grow. One school in Connecticut was so moldy that it had to be torn down.

Gail Bost, an AANMA outreach service coordinator from Franklin, Tennessee with an asthmatic teenage son, offered some excellent advice in the *MA Report* on improving air quality.

She initiated a pilot program for local schools using the "Indoor Air Quality Tools for Schools [IAQ TfS] Action Kit," which was developed by the Environmental Protection Agency (see www.epa.gov/iaq/schools). The program allows easy identification of problem areas, leading to low-cost strategies for many indoor air quality issues. The IAQ TfS kit includes a problem-solving wheel, renovation and repair checklists, a video on basic ventilation, and step-by-step instructions.

Says Ms. Bost, "Since implementing IAQ TfS, I've seen changes in teacher and staff attitudes at the school where I work. When the staff learned that room air fresheners contained harsh chemicals and that natural alternatives were available, the air fresheners disappeared. Our teachers are much more understanding and aware of what can cause problems for students with asthma."

The program has been such a success that it will be expanded into more schools.

How to proceed? Ms. Bost recommends creating a committee of teachers, staff, and parents, using surveys and discussions to learn about air quality in the school, and a committee walk-through of the

---

USEFUL WEBSITES FOR GOOD INFORMATION ABOUT ALLERGY AND SCHOOLS

www.aanma.org This site, created by Allergy & Asthma Network Mothers of Asthmatics, features the online town Breatherville, USA. Click on the school building to find information on keeping kids with asthma and allergies safe at school.

www.epa.gov/iaq/schools Learn more about the Environmental Protection Agency's "Indoor Air Quality Tools for Schools Action Kit," a resource that helps schools improve indoor air problems at little or no cost using straightforward activities and in-house staff.

www.lungusa.org Developed by the American Lung Association Asthma Friendly Schools Initiative, this educational site features a toolkit for planning "based on real-life activities that have been used in schools throughout the United States to create comprehensive asthma management systems."

www.healthyschools.org The Healthy Schools Network, Inc. advocates for environmentally healthy schools. Visit their site for tips on what you can do to clean up indoor environmental problems at your child's school or to purchase guides, fact sheets, and information packets. As a sign of the times, it includes guidelines for using federal stimulus funds to renovate schools in asthma-friendly ways, among other things.

www.allergy.org The Food Allergy & Anaphylaxis Network (FAAN) was established in 1991. FAAN's membership now stands at close to 30,000 worldwide and includes families, dietitians, nurses, physicians, school staff, and representatives from government agencies and the food and pharmaceutical industries. FAAN serves as the communications link between the patient and others. Click on teens/kids, schools/camps, and more. (continued on next page)

OTHER RESOURCES ABOUT ALLERGY AND SCHOOLS

• Asthma and Allergy Foundation of America: **www.aafa.org**
• Centers for Disease Control and Prevention:
www.cdc.gov/Features/ManageAsthma
• National Association of School Nurses: **www.nasn.org**.
Search keyword *asthma*.
• National Asthma Education and Prevention Program:
www.nhlbi.nih.gov/health/prof/lung/index.htm#asthma. Lists
numerous publications on every aspect of asthma awareness and
management in settings such as schools.
• National Education Association Health Information Network:
www.neahin.org. Search keyword *asthma*. 800-718-8387

---

school. It's important to remember that you can't fix every problem at once—continual follow-up is imperative.

Safety at Lunch

One New York City school had a nurse on duty—it's sad that a school should be considered fortunate to have a nurse—and three peanut-allergic students, all in kindergarten. Because each grade eats together, the nurse sits with them, EpiPens in hand, in case the dreaded peanuts migrate somehow. In a small, otherwise controlled setting, this is a way of letting kids be kids at lunch.

Change the School or Change Schools

According to Anne Muñoz-Furlong of FAAN, many schools are afraid of making themselves safe for food-allergic children because of liability issues, and 90 percent of them are parochial schools. They simply will not allow the child to attend. We mention this to warn you what you may encounter. Public schools can't be as choosy about which students come through their doors.

FAAN SCHOOL GUIDELINES FOR MANAGING STUDENTS WITH FOOD ALLERGIES

Food allergies can be life-threatening. The risk of accidental exposure to foods can be reduced in the school setting if schools work with students, parents, and physicians to minimize risks and provide a safe educational environment for food-allergic students.

Family's Responsibility

• Notify the school of the child's allergies.

• Work with the school team to develop a protocol that accommodates the child's needs throughout the school including in the classroom, in the cafeteria, in after-care programs, during school-sponsored activities, and on the school bus, as well as a Food Allergy Action Plan.

• Provide written medical documentation, instructions, and medications as directed by a physician, using the Food Allergy Action Plan as a guide. Include a photo of the child on the written form.

• Replace medications after use or upon expiration.

• Educate the child in the self-management of their food allergy including:

    Safe and unsafe foods

    Strategies for avoiding exposure to unsafe foods

    Symptoms of allergic reactions

    How and when to tell an adult they may be having an allergy-related problem

    How to read food labels (if age-appropriate)

• Review policies/procedures with school staff, the child's physician, and the child (if age-appropriate) after a reaction has occurred

School's Responsibility

• Be knowledgeable about and follow applicable federal laws including ADA, IDEA, Section 504, and FERPA, and any state laws or district policies that apply.

• Review the health records submitted by parents and physicians.

• Include food-allergic students in school activities. Students should not be excluded from school activities solely *(continued on next page)* based on their food allergy.

• Identify a core team including, but not limited to, school nurse, teacher, principal, school food service and nutrition manager/ director, and counselor (if available) to work with parents and the student (if age-appropriate) to establish a prevention plan. Changes to the prevention plan to promote food allergy management should be made with core team participation.

• Assure that any staff person who interacts with the student on a regular basis understands food allergy, can recognize symptoms, knows what to do in an emergency, and works with other school staff to eliminate the use of food allergens in the allergic student's meals, educational tools, arts-and-crafts projects, and incentives (such as food rewards for performance).

• Practice the Food Allergy Action Plans before an allergic reaction occurs, in order to assure the efficiency/effectiveness of the plans.

• Coordinate with the school nurse to be sure medications are appropriately stored, and be sure that an emergency kit is available that contains a physician's standing order for epinephrine. Keep the medications easily accessible in a secure location central to designated school personnel.

• Designate school personnel who are properly trained to administer medications in accordance with the State Nursing and Good Samaritan Laws governing the administration of emergency medications.

• Be prepared to handle a reaction. Ensure that there is a staff member available who is properly trained to administer medications during the school day, regardless of time or location.

• Review policies/prevention plan with the core team members, parents/guardians, student (if age-appropriate), and physician after a reaction has occurred.

• Work with the school district transportation administrator to assure that bus driver training includes symptom awareness and what to do if a reaction occurs.

• Recommend that all buses have communication devices in case of an emergency.

• Enforce a "no eating" policy on school buses, with exceptions made only to accommodate special needs under federal or other laws, or school district policy. Discuss *(continued on next page)* appropriate management of food allergy with family.

• Discuss field trips with the family of the food-allergic child to decide appropriate strategies for managing the food allergy.

• Follow federal/state/district laws and regulations regarding sharing medical information about the student.

• Take threats or harassment against an allergic child seriously.

Student's Responsibility

• Should not trade food with others.

• Should not eat anything with unknown ingredients or known to contain any allergen.

• Should be proactive in the care and management of their food allergies and reactions based on their developmental level.

• Should notify an adult immediately if they eat something they believe may contain the food to which they are allergic.

More detailed suggestions for implementing these objectives and creating a specific plan to address each individual student's particular needs are available in the Food Allergy & Anaphylaxis Network's (FAAN) School Food Allergy Program. This program has been endorsed and/or supported by the Anaphylaxis Committee of the American Academy of Allergy, Asthma & Immunology; the National Association of School Nurses; and the Executive Committee of the Section on Allergy and Immunology of the American Academy of Pediatrics. FAAN can be reached at 800-929-4040.

Guidelines were developed by the American School Food Service Association, National Association of Elementary School Principals, National Association of School Nurses, National School Boards Association, and the Food Allergy & Anaphylaxis Network.

A Summer at Camp

If schools are supermarkets of allergens, then summer camps are farms. Much of the traditional camp experience is defined by exposure to allergy triggers, from the leaf mold in the woods to the smoke from a campfire. Nowhere is the allergy paradox of primitive immunity provoked by the reality of modern life more starkly in evidence. We send our kids back to nature but nature itself is only tolerable if we send along a huge pharmacopoeia and an endless set of rules of conduct.

This is of course a great pity because camp is so much more than "nature." It is an escape from the heat and humidity of cities, and the cars, malls, and parents of the suburbs. It is a rite of passage, a chance to forge healthy independence from the structures of home and school, and to start on an equal social footing with a new set of peers—no cliques, clubs, or teams. It is a time to grow up. But not for kids with severe food allergies and especially not for asthmatics.

The father of one of our patients says,

"A few years ago, my wife and I were on an island off the Massachusetts coast when we got a call from the camp where all three of our children were staying. Our middle child—who had a history of mild asthma—and another asthmatic had attacks on an overnight. They were taken to the infirmary where many rounds of nebulizers did no good and they were taken to the hospital where they were stabilized. We had to clean the house, pack up, take a ferry to the mainland, and drive for six hours to the hospital with the vision of our little boy on the brink of death.

"This didn't do any of us any good. Did it mean some quantum leap in the seriousness of his condition? Did it mean he would never complete his childhood but always require the same level of trained personnel to be nearby? Would we parents always have to be on call?"

Unhappily for many families, the answer to all those questions has been "yes."

HORSEBACK RIDING FOR ASTHMATICS

- No camper may ride horses if known to be allergic to horses or other barnyard items such as hay.
- Campers must remove horse-riding clothing and bag in plastic before entering cabins.
- Campers must shower before returning to cabin.
- It would be prudent to keep campers who ride horses from bunking with campers who are allergic to horses.
- Have an albuterol inhaler with spacer available to the counselor leading the horseback riding activity.

What Can We Do About It?

Fortunately, a great deal. The growing prevalence of asthma has forced the camp industry to accommodate these children. Mainstream camps have been compelled to add asthma-safe protocols to their normal operations, which also include food allergy protections. And for those with even greater problems, there are growing numbers of camps that cater specifically to asthmatics. The website www.asthmacamps.org—operated by the Consortium on Children's Asthma Camps—not only lists such camps but provides all the information necessary to set up such a camp, including: how to make horseback riding safe for *some* asthmatics (see box); menus of activities; staff skill requirements, medical and nonmedical; and all the pharmaceuticals and paraphernalia needed to stock an infirmary.

Here is a list of medication and equipment to provide for emergencies on any trip away from the campsite.

MEDICATIONS

Acetaminophen

Albuterol inhaler

Albuterol inhalant solution

Hydroxyzine (Atarax)
25 mg PO

Diphenhydramine (Benadryl)
25 mg PO

Diphenhydramine (Benadryl)
25 mg IM

Chlorpheniramine 4 mg PO

Epinephrine 1:1,000 SQ (two)
(EpiPen—Jr and regular, preferred; Twinject)

Maalox tablets

Normal saline packets

Antibiotic ointment packets

Sudafed 30 mg tablets

Terbutaline 1 mg/ml SQ

Throat lozenges

Visine

EQUIPMENT

Stethoscope

Padlock and key
(in order to safeguard
all medicines!)

Peak flow meter and
mouthpieces

Water jug

Flashlight

Portable nebulizer

Nebulizer tubing

Nebulizer cups

Standing orders in plastic sleeve

Camper's charts in
waterproof pack

Of course, not every camp is guaranteed to be this thorough. In our practice, before our patients go away, we communicate with the camp administration about their procedures, medical capabilities (especially access to emergency care), and activities. While horseback riding can obviously be safe for some children, if we're not satisfied that the riding program measures up, we will veto it. One prohibition that grieves us is asking that kids be excused from certain chores, such as sweeping their bunks because stirring up dust will trigger an attack. In addition to providing children with recreational, social, and educational opportunities not available the other ten months of the year, camp teaches them how to clean up after themselves—surely an important lesson. We recommend, however, that camps detail these kids with other specified "character-building" activities.

CHAPTER 12

Allergies and the Environment

Environmental Diseases

A LLERGIES AND ASTHMA ARE, IN GREAT PART, ENVIRONMENTAL diseases. Allergens floating in the air are inhaled and lodge in the airways, provoking a response. The offending substances in allergens are usually made of proteins from such living things as the skin of animals, referred to as dander, dust, tiny insect parts, mold spores, and pollen. Some of these are perennial, around all the time, and some are seasonal, around only at certain parts of the year. For example, ragweed pollen, a major allergen, is only around in the late summer when the ragweed itself is flowering (although the season is longer in the South than in Northern states), and the air echoes with the sound of sneezing.

Newly mown grass is highly allergenic, so anyone who wants to instill a sense of responsibility in their children by assigning regular chores should try to find another task for kids with allergies. Cleaning the basement is probably not a good one either because of dust and molds.

Size and Allergens

A irborne allergens are small. They have to be small enough to make it into the nose and through a complex network of airways that get smaller the deeper you go. To trigger asthma, they have to be even smaller and get through an obstacle course of hair, mucus, and saliva before they are deposited in the bronchial airways. The different allergens vary in size. Large particles like mite dust settle into rugs and fly only for a short time into the air when disturbed, while the smaller particles of cat dander can stay in the air for long periods and travel far.

WHEN THE BOMB DROPS

During the Cold War, I was a student allergist working on a study of ragweed allergy injections with a group of scientists at Johns Hopkins. We needed to know the ragweed pollen count. At that time, allergists counted ragweed by the gravity method. A microscope slide was placed outside and the number of pollen grains falling in 24 hours was counted. A scientist pointed out the number of grains on the slide did not accurately reflect what was in the air because of wind currents.

I was dispatched after security clearance to an atomic research center. They were growing ragweed in a circular patch and studying how the pollen spread out as a model of what would happen to the radioactive particles coming from an atomic bomb blast.

Being physicists, they had designed a better counter than the allergist's gravity slide, one that spun around in circles to cancel the effects of wind currents. This rotoslide pollen counter is now standard.
— *Dr. Chiaramonte*

Geography Matters

We are exposed to these allergens constantly both indoors and outside. If the air is completely free of the substances an allergic patient is sensitive to, there will be no symptoms. If someone is dust sensitive, for example, and moves to the top of the Swiss Alps where the air is very clean, cold, and dry, her allergic symptoms will disappear. Similarly, if a cat-sensitive asthmatic gives away his cat, his asthma often improves dramatically.

Allergenic proteins are entirely harmless in and of themselves, and cause no reaction in about 80 percent of the American population. This doesn't seem fair: A dog is a man's best friend but may be his child's greatest nuisance.

Allergens responsible for allergy vary from residence to residence and from region to region. For example, cockroaches are a very important cause of asthma among inner-city populations, while in the mountain states, cats and dogs cause more allergy. Molds have been reported to be the dominant asthma-related allergens both in the humid Pacific Northwest, and in dry areas like Arizona where they grow in the water of cooling systems. One thing all these allergies have in common is the discomfort and misery they cause.

The four major indoor allergens in the United States are dust mites, cockroaches, pet dander, and mold spores. In vermin-infested homes, mouse and rat allergens may be involved. Pollen and mold spores are the major outdoor allergens responsible for seasonal asthma. Let's take them individually.

Dust Mites

Dust mites are the most important indoor allergens in many areas of the world. Many millions of people suffer from allergic rhinitis and other allergic conditions because of them. In addition, they were identified as a cause of asthma almost thirty years ago and today, 60 to 80 percent of patients with asthma throughout the world are allergic to dust mites.

Dust mites are microscopic, spiderlike insects. Their main source of food is the skin that humans shed at the rate of about one gram per week for adults. This dead skin accumulates in carpets, mattresses, and upholstered furniture and constitutes the major component of house dust. Mites only need three things to survive: a source of food, i.e, human skin, which explains their scientific name, *Dermatophagoides*, meaning "skin eater" in Greek; moisture (generally humidity greater than 50 percent); and a warm temperature (about 70°F).

What's the warmest, dampest, and most skin-filled place in the home? The bed, which is why the bed is "dust mite central" in most homes. Our children spend eight hours or more a night wallowing in it.

The most allergenic component of dust mites is their feces. The particles are the same size and shape as pollen grains so they are easily inhaled and drawn into the bronchial airways. Every ounce of dust in a mattress contains about a quarter of a million fecal pellets, courtesy of mites. Therefore, most individuals in the developed world spend about eight hours every night breathing the stuff. The more dust-mite allergen, the more likely asthma will develop. About 23 percent of American homes have dust-mite allergen levels high enough to cause asthma. They know no social distinction; their presence in a home is determined by temperature and humidity, not social class.

Animal Allergens

Approximately 70 percent of American households have one or more pets. Cats are the most common and cat dander is the most common cause of asthma. Dander does not come from hair or skin itself, but comes from a protein produced by sweat glands.

As cats lick their fur, they coat themselves with a fine layer of this allergen, which dries and floats off into the air, producing the cloud of allergens that constantly envelops most cats. Unlike mite allergens, which are heavy and settle to the ground, cat-dander allergens can remain airborne for long periods of time. They are also very sticky and cling to wall surfaces and clothing. When a pet owner's clothing touches clothing of non–pet owners—in a schoolroom coat closet, for example—allergens move from one to another and are carried back to homes with no cats.

The idea that a breed can be "hypoallergenic" received a great deal of publicity when then President-elect Barack Obama listed his

---

THE CASE OF THE INVISIBLE CATS

In the winter of 1974 the energy prices soared three- to fourfold. Naturally, the reaction to the crisis was to look for ways to save energy, permanently if possible, by upgrading the efficiency of our infrastructure. We built public buildings that conserved energy. Schools in particular built at this time allowed for little exchange of indoor air with the outdoor environment, making them allergy prone by reducing the natural cleansing effect of ventilation on indoor air.

Twelve-year-old Joe tells us, "I do not like school, because I could being doing other fun things, but I want to get into a good college. It is just every time I go to school I feel like I am with a cat. I become itchy all over, my eyes turn red, and I start to sneeze my head off."

Smart boy, that Joe. Although there were no cats at school, naturally, several of his classmates had cats. Their coats were in a nearby room with little air exchange with the outdoors. These coats with their cat dander were enough to trigger Joe's sensitive allergies. That is why cat allergens can be found in the dust and air of homes that have never had pets, and why elementary school classrooms spread pet allergy so effectively.

---

daughter Malia's allergies as one criterion the family would consider in choosing the White House dog. The family eventually settled on a Portuguese water dog, a breed that has a reputation for being hypoallergenic, primarily because they do not shed. The same is true for poodles.

However, cats and dogs that are advertised as "hypoallergenic" are probably a myth since the allergens of all mammals of the same species are similar. The pet's type of hair, fur length, or sex does not make it more or less allergenic. On the other hand, the size and behavior of an animal and grooming habits of the owner do affect the quantity of allergen it will produce. Large dogs such as German shepherds can give off as much as a hundred times more allergen than small ones, such as Chihuahuas. Pets that go everywhere in a home and onto the furniture cause more allergy than those that stay outside or are kept in one room. Pet owners who allow their pets into the bedroom, especially onto the bed, are at the greatest risk for developing severe asthma. Frequent pet baths can considerably reduce the quantity of allergen.

However, if genome researchers ever succeed in breeding a truly non-allergenic cat, they will surely make a fortune.

All other mammals, such as rodents, rabbits, and farm animals, shed dander and can trigger asthma. As with cats and dogs, size and behavior determine how much of a problem they present. People often report that they are allergic to other pets but not to their own. They may not have acute symptoms when they are around their pets, so they mistakenly assume that their pets are not the cause of their asthma. In fact, they are very likely suffering from chronic inflammation at a level they are accustomed to, but it can be pushed over the threshold into an attack outside the home. This may be because they have come into contact with someone else's pet, but the real culprit may also be some unseen environmental element, such as mold or high levels of dust.

These same patients often find that their asthma worsens when they return after an extended period of time away from home, on a vacation, say, or off at college. This suggests that they were always allergic to their pet but had become tolerant of the symptoms. When a patient left home and experienced less chronic inflammation, re-exposure to little Mittens sparked a reaction.

Feathers are often overlooked as a source of allergy. Of course they are on birds but can be present in the home and other environments even when there are no birds—in pillows, for example, and sometimes on costumes.

Mary Jo was a patient who came to me with severe allergic rhinitis and stated that she was worse at her job. What made this most interesting was that she worked as an ecdysiast—a.k.a. stripper—in a Times Square joint (back in the days when Times Square was a less Disneyfied place). She said she enjoyed her work, but sneezed like crazy as she got further along in her act. She complained that although the men in the front row loved the pronounced effects on certain parts of her body when she sneezed, she had a hard time keeping in step with the music. Periodically she would blow her nose in a discrete fashion, but by the end of the act, "I had no place to keep my Kleenex."

This was in the days before the Americans with Disabilities Act, so there was no relief available to Mary Jo from a legal point of view for a workplace disability. However, it was also in the days before our current health insurance crisis took hold, so I undertook a comprehensive approach to her plight. Testing revealed a severe sensitivity to house dust and feathers. Being the professional that I am, I made several calls to her place of work in order to observe firsthand these deplorable conditions. This was scientific dedication at its best.

Dust was a persistent backstage problem and there was little that could be done about it, but the feathers were an artistic one and art is about nothing if not choice. May Jo discarded her feathers and her colleagues were good enough to follow suit. In addition, immunotherapy worked well, although we had to be inventive in finding sites for her injections that would not redound to her artistic detriment.

— *Dr. Ehrlich*

Cockroaches

Cockroaches are a very significant cause of asthma. They are common in multiple-family dwellings in most major U.S. cities, including expensive apartment buildings, as well as in single-family homes in warm, humid parts of the country. It is estimated that one visible roach represents a population of a hundred roaches living in the walls. Many parts of the cockroach are allergenic, including their bodies, urine, feces, and saliva. When they die, their bodies break down and they become part of the house dust. In old apartment buildings, there may be many years' roach allergen in the dust, so anyone living in a home where there have been roaches at any time is at risk.

While roach allergen concentration is highest in the kitchen, the bedroom is a more important venue for exposure simply because we spend so much time in it. An estimated 6 million U.S. bedrooms contain enough cockroach allergen to cause asthma.

LESSON LEARNED—
KNOW YOUR PATIENT'S ENVIRONMENT

Almost thirty years ago we were treating asthmatic children from the poor areas of Brooklyn. The children had a resistant form of asthma compared to the middle-class children I was treating in Queens. Why?

The standard answer from allergists who only worked in upscale areas was that these poor patients and parents were too dumb or too lazy to follow instructions. Our controlled study proved otherwise. When we asked them to do something within their resources, it was done as well if not better than in middle-class homes.

In another controlled study, we tested for allergens in the group from middle-class, single-family homes and the clinic group from high-rise apartments. We added nontraditional allergens—cockroach, mice, and rats. The clinic group from Brooklyn was positive to these "inner-city allergens" and their asthma seemed to improve more rapidly when we began treating for these allergens. In the mid-1970s we published these findings but they seemed to have little impact; Brooklyn as a research venue carried little weight in those days.

In the 1990s a study at Johns Hopkins in Baltimore on poor, inner-city children failed to show that allergy immunotherapy worked. We and others pointed out that the injections did not contain cockroach antigen. When the study was repeated on children from the Bronx with cockroach antigen, they were shown to be effective.

— *Dr. Chiaramonte*

Molds (Fungi)

Molds are widespread in the environment and are common causes of severe allergies and asthma. Molds are a primitive type of plant. Their spores are similar in size to pollen grains. Some common molds are visible, such as the blue mold that grows on stale bread and cheese or the black mildew between your bathroom tiles. Molds grow inside homes wherever it is moist, such as in damp basements and around leaky plumbing. Like pollen grains, the mold spores themselves are microscopic so most molds cannot be seen. But you can smell them! Thus, a nonallergic person knows when he is entering a room with mildew because of the musty smell. The person with allergic rhinitis, however, will not only smell it, but will feel like the

---

DON'T BLAME NEW JERSEY

I treated a boy whose fairly affluent family moved from an apartment in a nice Brooklyn neighborhood to a new house in a New Jersey suburb. Before they left, his asthma was well controlled, but after a couple of weeks in the new home, it returned with a vengeance. After emergency intervention and some frantic calls to me, I admonished the mother to find someplace else for the child to stay to get some relief and give us time to sort the problem out. She was able to move them into her mother's house and the child showed immediate improvement. After five days, they returned to the house, and once again the symptoms returned.

I told her to have an engineer inspect the house, and he reported the startling information that some of the flashing—sheet metal installed at the junction of roofs, chimneys, walls, windows, and other places where one building material meets another—had been installed backwards. Every time it rained, instead of deflecting water away from the house, it was channeled back into the walls, where mold was now rampant.

My snobby New York neighbors draw one message from this— that people should know better than to move to New Jersey. But the real lesson is that when a disease like asthma appears, you have to look everywhere for clues.

In this case, there was no real way to medicate asthma out of this child's life. His family had to move.

— *Dr. Ehrlich*

---

inside of his nose is being tickled.

Outdoor mold levels are highest when it is warm and humid: June to October in most parts of the U.S., and mold-allergic asthmatics often have worse symptoms during these times. Take care on those camping vacations!

However, dry weather conditions do not eliminate the possibility of mold exposure since some important outdoor molds predominate during dry weather, especially when it is windy.

Houses that are prone to mold can be painted with a product like Caliwel, which has been approved by the EPA to kill molds on contact. It is applied like any paint and can be active for up to six years, although contractors of our acquaintance are dubious of this claim.

Toxic Molds

There have been many reports in the news regarding toxic molds and their products, known as mycotoxins. The cable TV show *Forensic Files* devoted an episode to a family beset with terrible neurological difficulties eventually traced to molds in their Texas McMansion.

Some molds such as *Stachybotrys chartarum*, *Fusarium*, and *Trichoderma* can produce very toxic compounds, which, when inhaled or ingested, may result in a poisoning known as mycotoxicosis, which is marked by respiratory, neurological, flu-like, gastrointestinal, and skin problems. These molds are rather uncommon and not every species produces toxins. Therefore, finding these molds does not mean that they actually are producing a toxin or causing mycotoxicosis. Deadly disease due to inhalation of mold toxins is probably rare.

Pollens

Pollen grains are microscopic particles produced by most plants and transported to other plants of the same species for reproduction. They are the plant equivalent of sperm. Only plants with pollen that is light and not sticky, and can therefore be spread by the wind, are common causes of asthma. Unfortunately this includes many species of trees, grasses, and weeds. In order to success-fully transmit their pollen to other members of their species, trees, grasses, and weeds produce enormous amounts of pollen that can be blown upwards of fifty miles and can be detected as high in the air as the Empire State Building. It is these windborne pollens that are reported daily as pollen counts and cause major problems for allergic asthmatics.

Most plants with colorful, perfumed flowers, by contrast, produce heavy, sticky pollen grains that cling to the legs of bees and other insects and generally do not cause major asthma problems. With some flowering plants, their pollen is no threat but they may be allergenic when eaten. Such is the case with the sunflower depicted on the cover of this book.

There is a well-defined seasonal pollen cycle. In the Northern U.S., tree pollen appears early in the spring, before the leaves unfold. Grass pollen appears later in the spring and early summer. Finally, there is a late summer peak of weeds and ragweed. Hay fever is named for the period when grasses mature and are mown for hay, although the pollens may have nothing to do with agriculture. In warmer areas of the U.S., such as the Southeast or Southern California, the grass season may last six months or more. Also, areas such as Southern California, much of which is essentially desert, are devoid of ragweed, and do not have a hay-fever season.

Depending on what pollens they are allergic to, asthmatics may have increased symptoms during different times of the pollen season. For example, in New York City, there is an increase in asthma emer-gency room visits in the spring, a short time after the peak in tree pollen, as well as another smaller asthma spike in the late summer, about two weeks after the ragweed peak. Activity picks up again in October and November because of atmospheric inversions, molds from falling leaves, and dust blowing around inside buildings when heating systems are turned on.

The relationship between allergen exposure and allergic symp-toms is a little like drinking and getting drunk. The first drink or allergen exposure does not do much but more drinks or allergen expo-sure will bring more trouble more easily. Finally there is a hangover effect: Allergic symptoms and being drunk persists even after allergen exposure or drinking has stopped.

NOTHING TO SNEEZE AT

The world of allergic medicine is confused by conventional wisdom and folklore, as explained here in the seminal 1935 text *Pollen Grains* by botanist Roger P. Wodehouse, who first observed and illustrated the pollens of many flowers:

"The expression, late summer hayfever, will call to the minds of many the goldenrods, sunflowers, and other gorgeous components of the waning summer's landscape, for the impression that these flowers must be the cause of their malady has become deeply fixed with many whose sufferings are ushered in with the appearance of such flowers. The term 'goldenrod fever' has been popularly suggested to describe the form of hayfever occurring when the goldenrods bloom but only with the justification of coincidence in time."

Occupational Allergens

While occupational allergens are not an immediate cause of concern for children, it bears thinking about them for a number of reasons. For example, children visit their parents' workplaces. Then, too, there's the chance that they might go into a profession some day where they are likely to be exposed to a wide range of airborne substances that can cause allergies and asthma. These include such things as laboratory animal dander, grain and flour dust that affect bakers and agricultural workers, other foodstuffs such as coffee bean dust, dust from woods such as mahogany or western red cedar, and chemicals like platinum or toluene diisocyanate that affect people who spray paint. Substances like psyllium, which is found in laxatives like Metamucil, can cause asthma in those who handle large amounts of the powder, such as nurses and pharmacists.

Exposure to latex gloves has become a common problem among health care workers, and is likely to present a problem to children who do laboratory experiments in school. Latex is made from the sap of the rubber tree and the gloves may contain residual amounts of plant protein, which becomes airborne. When the gloves are powdered with starch to make them easier to use, the allergenic proteins stick to the powder, spreading it further and making powdered gloves more likely to cause asthma than nonpowdered ones. Powder-free, low-protein gloves are much less allergenic and should be used exclusively by latex-sensitive individuals if nonlatex gloves are not available.

Interestingly, latex-sensitive individuals are often allergic to a variety of other fruits and vegetables, such as kiwi, avocado, and banana, which, like latex, also happen to be grown in tropical climes.

Other Indoor Airborne Irritants

In addition to allergens, indoor air often contains irritating substances that irritate allergies. Secondhand tobacco smoke is probably the most common. Others include chemical fumes from paint, insecticides, smoke from wood stoves, fumes from scented candles, and even perfume. Gas stoves give off nitrogen dioxide, a known respiratory irritant. Asthmatics in poorly ventilated homes will experience more symptoms when such stoves are used, especially if they are used as an extra source of heating during the winter.

Home Environmental Allergen Reduction

Because allergens are so important in causing asthma, the single most effective measure asthmatics can take is to reduce their exposure to allergens whenever possible. The most practical place to do this is in the home where the first goal should be to reduce dust levels in the bedroom. Many studies have demonstrated significant improvements in asthma after bedroom dust is removed. In fact, the bedroom should be as free as possible from all known and potential asthma triggers regardless of evidence of allergies.

The biggest mistake patients make is to assume it is acceptable to sleep with their cat, or to continue using a feather pillow because they were told that they were not allergic. Denial plays a heavy part in the failure to take sound measures to reduce home allergens. We hear excuses like "my cat never bothered me before" or "I slept with a feather pillow before I developed asthma." But prior exposure is the essence of allergic disease. It may take a long period of exposure to allergens to make someone allergic, but having lived for long periods without symptoms does not mean the allergens are not causing problems.

SLEEP ALLERGY FREE

All surroundings of the dust-sensitive patient should be as free as possible from any dust. This is the single most important step in treatment of asthma and allergies. Do as much as you can, since anything you do will be helpful.

Step 1. Pets — Remove any furry or feathered animals from the bedroom, permanently. No pets should ever be in the bedroom, even when the patient is not there.

Step 2. Bedding — Discard any feather (or down) pillows or quilts. Use hypoallergenic (polyester) pillows and washable blankets. Blankets should be washed immediately and often to keep them dust free.

Step 3. Heating and air-conditioning — Forced-air ventilation is very bad for patients. Buy filter material (Vent-Gard or equivalent) and install in the bedroom air-inlet vent, so that all the air that enters the room is filtered. Wash or change this filter every month.

Step 4. Humidifiers — Do not use humidifiers of any kind. Increased humidity increases the growth of dust mites and molds and will make you worse. The most effective way to keep your air passages comfortable during the night is to keep the bedroom very cold (55°F –60°F).

Step 5. Plastic covers — The patient's bed must have plastic covers that completely encase any pillows, the mattress, and box spring. Do this even if the mattress and pillows are new.

Step 6. Rugs — Remove any rugs and carpets. All rugs trap dust whether they are wool or synthetics. Hardwood or vinyl floors are preferable but a washable throw rug can be used. If it is impossible to remove carpeting, vigorous vacuuming must be performed daily.

Step 7. Vacuum cleaners — Vacuum cleaners blow a lot of fine dust out the back. Purchase special allergen-proof vacuum cleaner bags. Special vacuum cleaners such as the Miele or Nilfisk work well, but are very expensive.

Step 8. HEPA air purifiers — HEPA air purifiers are very useful when there are allergens floating *(continued on next page)* in the air in your bedroom, such as pet dander, mold spores, or cigarette smoke, or if you have forced-air ventilation. They can run all the time, but only when the door and windows are closed.

Step 9 General clean up and other dust collectors — Remove all upholstered furniture, drapes, old books and newspapers, and stuffed animals. Wooden or metal chairs and plain light curtains can be used. Clean the woodwork and floors to remove all traces of dust.

Step 10. Regular cleaning — The room must be cleaned daily and given a thorough and complete cleaning once a week. Clean the floors, furniture, tops of doors, window frames, sills, etc. with a damp cloth. Air the room thoroughly but keep the door of this room closed as much as possible. Remember, the cleaner the room, the better the patient will feel.

The same rules should be applied throughout the house. In addition, any source of indoor moisture can be a source of mold growth and should be eliminated. Mold spores can be effectively removed by regular ventilation and washing affected areas with household bleach. Indoor humidity should be maintained at 50 percent or lower by using air conditioning and dehumidifiers. Sump pumps should be used in damp or flooded basements.

Cockroach Eradication

Cockroach removal presents a problem that is often very difficult to solve, especially in inner-city, multifamily dwellings. The bedroom allergen elimination measures described above will help, but roach infestation from the rest of the house must be halted in order to remove a constant source of new allergen. The most important measure is to remove all sources of food and water that sustain roach populations. Food should be kept in tightly sealed glass jars or plastic tubs, or kept in the refrigerator. Dishes should be washed immediately after use and not left in the sink. Pet food should be left out only for short periods of time, and kitty litter should be changed every few days. Washing all surfaces with soap daily, vacuuming under furniture, and removing clutter will help. All holes and cracks should be sealed and caulked and any leaky plumbing should be repaired. Trash must be emptied daily and garbage cans should have lids and plastic bag inserts that tie on top.

The use of safe insecticides is essential for eliminating roaches. Gel baits or bait stations are the safest and most effective method of treating asthmatic homes. It is important to place these not only in the kitchen but also in the bedroom, out of the reach of children and pets. Baits must be changed every three months to remain effective and other insecticides should not be used at the same time. Insect sprays or pesticide bombs, which can exacerbate asthma, should be avoided.

NOWHERE TO HIDE

When I was in training to be an allergist at a New York hospital, an industrialist who had allergies gave us the money to build an allergen-free room. He had used the new "clean room technology" in his business and was convinced he could treat allergy by putting asthmatics in this room. At best we got only mixed results. The asthmatics would live in this room for a few days. Allergens such as molds, mites, and foods were present even though the air was constantly filtered. — *Dr. Chiaramonte*

Stirring Up Trouble

Allergy is a tough field. Symptoms can overlap with those from nonallergic disease, complicating diagnosis and treatment. Large-scale exposures to particulates, such as diesel fumes, and chemicals released by building demolition, up to and including the collapse of the World Trade Center, can exacerbate allergic and asthmatic tendencies. Treatment can involve most of the same protocols that we describe in the pages of this book. When something as serious as 9/11 happens, there may be no long-term cure, even though the exposure may not last very long.

The bigger problem for large numbers of children and adults is that the exposure may not be as acute, but it goes on and on, such as diesel and industrial matter that is concentrated in poor urban neighborhoods, like the ones your authors practice in regularly. Mere economics is no guarantee of safety, as there are "asthma corridors" even in richer neighborhoods.

The *New York Times* (Dec. 17, 2009) wrote that the Upper East Side of Manhattan, which has some of the country's wealthier zip codes, has some of the city's filthiest air. In addition to vehicular traffic, the boilers in the basements of distinguished older buildings burn heavier oil than newer burners, resulting in higher concentrations of particulates and sulfur dioxide.

Rural areas, too, are prone to problems from industrial-scale agriculture, especially around manure lagoons that capture waste from feedlots and dairies. The lungs and sinuses of allergy and asthma patients who live near the pollution sources are in perpetual red alert. A renewed emphasis on clean air would help the health of millions of Americans.

As with food allergies, however, it's often difficult to figure out where allergies end and other physical disease begins. The prevalence of chemicals in our environment confuses the issues.

For example, there is something called MCS (multiple chemical sensitivity), a term coined a couple of decades ago by Dr. Mark Cullen, then head of the Occupational Medicine department at Yale (now Chief of General Internal Medicine at Stanford), to describe a variety of symptoms that stem from alterations in a person's indoor environment, primarily at work, but sometimes at home. So-called "sick building syndrome" may be caused by chemicals in modern building materials, or it may be a function of ventilation problems caused by new construction methods and energy-saving techniques. Unless new air is exchanged for old air at a certain rate, allergens, toxins, or chemical residue can become concentrated at levels high enough to provoke a reaction. The problem seemed to coincide with the creation of new building codes written after the energy crisis of the 1970s, when engineers felt they could save energy by recirculating air that had already been heated or cooled, instead of bringing in new air from the outside. Just as problematic is the process of renovation, when molds, mouse droppings, dust, or chemicals that have been undisturbed may be stirred up and circulate in the building.

The good news for parents is that MCS seems to be a problem for the middle-aged, not for children. People are more likely to encounter it when they change jobs or move to a new workplace than their kids are. Still, whether the worry is chemicals or such proven allergens as molds and mouse droppings, there is always a chance that they will activate their children's plain old allergies in the event they renovate their homes, or if a child's school is going to be renovated.

We therefore advise that:

• Children be isolated from renovation activity, especially during the demolition phase of construction.

• When the old materials are stripped out, the exposed areas be inspected for water damage, and that all areas be thoroughly swept for vermin residue, dust, and so forth.

• Your architect incorporate the requisite specifications for healthy air exchange.

• Any central heating and cooling system be easy to maintain and clean, to discourage buildup of viruses and toxic bacteria.

Likewise, if your child's school is planning an overhaul, consult with school officials to ensure that the children's health is provided for.

CHAPTER 13

Allergic Children Are Children, Too

THE MOST IMPORTANT THING TO REMEMBER ABOUT YOUR allergic child is that she or he is a child. Allergies complicate childhood but don't necessarily change it. Allergic children do the same developmentally appropriate things nonallergic children do. They may be uncomfortable or sick more often than other children. They may be depressed, frustrated, or angry as a result of their allergies. But to the extent that we can treat them effectively and endeavor mightily to give them the same kind of childhood enjoyed by their less-encumbered peers, they can get through it and eventually "outgrow" their allergies, psychologically if not physically.

Without a doubt, the effects of allergy, particularly food allergy, can be both subtle and substantial. Sally Noone, who conducts clinical food allergy studies at Mount Sinai Hospital in New York City, says that she was drawn into the field by the case of a girl who was hospitalized after a milk-allergy attack at the age of 4. This little girl, despite the success of her parents at insulating her from further such exposures, became phobic about food several years later, even with the lunches that her mother packed for her to take to school. It took psychotherapy to overcome her difficulties.

Terrible Twos and Up

Experienced as the two of us are, we don't presume to be able to get into the heads of preverbal children, although many do have allergies such as colic, eczema, allergic eyes, and so on. However, treating kids for allergy is complicated by the same stages of development that all normal children have. For example, it is normal for a child—or anyone else—to scratch an itch, and this can lead to a visible outbreak, eczema. It is the allergy to, say, milk that makes her itch, which we can't see, but she can feel. The thickened scaly skin we associate with eczema is really the result of itching. Her own nails can infect her skin with superficial staph bacteria when she scratches, causing weeping open or crusted sores. This is why "eczema" often responds to antibiotics, although many doctors treat it with other means. There is a medical aphorism, "Eczema is an itch in search of a rash." The allergist's job would be to treat the itch.

Treating a child between the ages of 2 and 3 is different from treating a child between 3 and 4. Why? Because one is in that very real stage known as the "terrible twos," when children say no to everything and begin to test their debating skills, whereas by the time four rolls around, they are more likely to have reached an age of (comparative) reason. Up to the time of preadolescence, children seem to attain some degree of ease with their treatment. They become knowledgeable and even cooperative, although boys and girls are somewhat different. They remain reasonable until they approach adolescence, when a whole new set of dynamics kick in, and the gender differences become more pronounced.

At each stage, the reaction to allergy treatment is going to track the ongoing saga of passage towards adulthood.

The Anxiety of the Allergic Child

Sadly, we must point out that even very young patients occasionally come to us in a fairly anxious or depressed state. This is not only because they may be suffering considerable discomfort, but also because their moods are colored by those of their parents, who may be suffering feelings of guilt, anxiety, and helplessness. A toddler with bad eczema has not only been itching like crazy, but his parents have been obsessing about the rash, and the pediatrician has been trying every remedy under the sun. In our experience, it is at the point of despair that the pediatrician hands the child off to a pediatric allergist—not the worst thing in the world from our point of view but bad for the parents and child.

Once that child arrives in our office, he has very likely built up some real baggage of his own. He sits there listening to his mother obsess about his misery and that of everyone else at home. He feels resentment from his siblings for attracting so much attention. He feels guilty for causing trouble and feels scared that he will never get better. In that fraught atmosphere, the doctor must not only gain the child's confidence, but look in his ears, listen to his chest, and even give him shots.

DR. CHIARAMONTE'S KIDDIE CASE FILE

Joking Around

"What is the matter, Chrissy? Why are you crying?" I asked the 4-year-old girl.

"It is that *teethoscope*—you know what I mean—it is cold and I do not like dentists."

"Why don't you try it on me?" I say, putting the earpieces in her ears and the diaphragm on my chest. "Do you hear my heart beating?" She finally smiled and nodded yes.

"Now please tell me when it stops?"

She got the joke and let me listen to her chest.

Tough Guy

Tough Tony from Brooklyn, a 13-year-old with muscles beyond his years shouted, "I don't care how small the needles are, you're not giving me a shot, and if you try I'll take that stethoscope and wrap it around your neck."

"Oh yeah?!"—all vestiges of my Ivy League education disappearing. "How about this?" I pulled out a *3-liter* syringe we used for checking our lung-function machine—one that's about three feet long.

Tough Tony turned pale, looked at me, and then suddenly smiled. "OK," he said, "You got me. You win."

Let's Make a Deal

Some kids are born negotiators and sometimes we have to incorporate that into treatment. One big advantage of being an experienced allergist is that you know from the history which tests are important to administer and which ones aren't. Whereas a GP might order a full battery of eighteen scratch tests just to be on the safe side, the pediatric allergist will only be interested in four or five. So if the child says he doesn't want any tests, you can start with a high bid and let him negotiate you down to the number you wanted anyway. This gives the child a sense of power over his own medical condition that has been lacking.

— *Dr. Chiaramonte*

We are, of course, both pediatric allergists, and without sounding too smug about our own subspecialty, there's a good reason to go to a pediatric allergist for your child, not just a regular adult allergist. Apart from the differences in the way the allergic diseases present themselves at different ages, and the way they should be treated, there's the matter of what we might call "crib-side manner." That is, we try to relate to the child as close to his own terms as we can. This gives us a chance to become children again if just for a moment. We have to love doing this or it will show. Because of our training and because of our frequent collaboration with pediatricians we have tricks up our sleeves to gain the confidence of both parents and children that make difficult, annoying treatment go more smoothly.

An important "trick" we have in the office is doing whatever has to be done to Mom, Dad, or even ourselves first. Shot? We have the parents roll up their sleeves and give them a shot of saline. Or a dummy scratch test. We might use our stethoscope on Dad's chest or Mom's back to put the child at ease, or allow the child to listen to ours.

Why Allergic Life Gets Harder

Life gets harder for all children as they approach adolescence. Children are wrenched from the stability of elementary schools and their familiar classmates and thrown together with children from other schools. Middle schools have a reputation for being the lost years of education anyway, and in troubled school systems they are notoriously resistant to reform, so there's no guarantee that the new environment will be a happy one.

For all kids as they get older, there's a lot of experimentation with greater freedom from parental supervision, which might include unsupervised consumption of junk foods, different attitudes towards members of the opposite sex, and defiance of authority. Then there are all those glandular changes, which affect moods generally as well as libido. Kids who were once fairly equal in size and appearance separate into different groupings by shape, height, facial and body hair, and so on.

The allergic child is subject to all these adjustments and dislocations. But on top of the universal problems, the allergic child faces some special challenges. For example, after years in which his parents may have battled to create an allergy-safe environment in the elementary school, there's a whole new school to adjust to, and new children and staff to educate—not that the child wants Mom to come in and do that all over again.

Pre-adolescence and adolescence, moreover, are times when pressure to fit in is enormous. Allergies make a child different just when he doesn't want to be. He doesn't want to sit by himself in the lunchroom when everyone else is sitting with others. If a school is lucky enough to have a comprehensive physical-education program, there are damp, possibly moldy locker rooms to cope with and the possible embarrassment of communal changing and showering. Boys don't want to look frail or unathletic or "undeveloped" compared to others. They are more likely than girls to hide their metered-dose inhalers from their peers. They don't want to be embarrassed by fussing over special food when their friends blithely lunch on ice cream cones covered with chocolate and peanuts.

Then there are the "other" glandular adjustments besides the sexual ones. Of particular importance for allergy, the lymphoid system—the tonsils and lymph nodes—peaks at around the age of 12. Since the lymphoids influence the immune system, when they stop developing, it can't help but have an effect on the functioning of the immune system. The immune system continues to function but the levels and patterns of how it functions is set. Allergies seem to abate in 30–50 percent of teenage boys only to return in some after 40. Girls seem to have the onset of allergy in the late teens.

Temptation Outside School

Outside school, children are developing new, more independent social lives, which makes it harder and harder to police their diet. When they are with their peers at coffee shops and malls they will be tempted by easy access to ice cream and other possibly *verboten* foods. If their friends are ordering sundaes, who's to say that they may not put peanuts on them, even if they risk accidental exposure? They don't want to be the one kid at the confirmation parties or Bar Mitzvahs who never gets to eat and always has to watch out for what others have eaten. These feelings of strangeness can cause a lonely period of life to be even lonelier, although there are always those who feel special—usually girls—because they get to carry medicine with them.

While we want people to treat allergic children as "normal," the stresses and strains can have consequences if not tackled forthrightly. However, even the awkward moments can be handled with imagination, turning a challenge into a triumph.

WHEN LIFE HANDS YOU A LEMON, MAKE LEMONADE

I had one patient who was coming up for his Bar Mitzvah. He had gone to many Bar Mitzvahs for his friends and refrained from eating because he was allergic to milk, wheat, and eggs.

"Dr. Ehrlich how can I have fun at my Bar Mitzvah with my food allergies? I am to become a man but I am not in control of the menu," moaned David.

"Well, I guess we can work out a menu. We want you to become a man." Of course, my imagination in this area was limited by my own cooking skills.

"Wait a minute," he said. You could almost see the light bulb going on over his head. "How about a cooking school, where my friends and I could be creative with our own recipes without the allergic foods?"

Listen, listen to your patients and you will learn.

Sure enough, his parents located such a cooking school and made the arrangements. It was a tremendous hit. Even the boys wore aprons. He became a minor celebrity because it was the most interesting Bar Mitzvah party anyone had ever been to. *— Dr. Ehrlich*

Teenagers

Life gets still more difficult in high school. This is a time when those loving little people turn into what the novelist Alison Lurie called "big strangers." They may live in your home, but they are not the kids you once knew. If you're lucky, the little ones will return as loving as ever, with all their good childhood traits intact, but all grown up. With allergic or asthmatic children, the natural pulling away and assertion of independent identity are compromised by the illness. The EpiPen or inhaler they have to carry with them are like Mom's apron strings. Dietary limitations and discipline are like having the old lady looking over their shoulders while they are out driving around with friends and going through other rites of passage. The parents of nonallergic friends "only" have to worry about driving, drinking, and drugs. The parents of allergic children get to worry about ice cream and peanuts as well as cigarette smoking and their friends' pets.

And with good reason. The "I'm going to live forever" teenage exuberance is a well-known and sometimes tragic impulse. It prompts so many to flirt with disaster when they get behind the wheel of a car or get a phony ID to let them buy beer. And it has its own analog among allergic and asthmatic teenagers who get careless or even defiant about taking medications and avoiding allergens.

Over the years, Sally Noone of Mount Sinai has run many discussion groups for adolescents about their allergy and asthma under the auspices of the Food Allergy & Anaphylaxis Network (FAAN). These are, admittedly, the most informed children of the most informed adults so they are not representative of every child with asthma. Still, because a high degree of allergy consciousness is present in these kids, they represent our best opportunity to study the normal child lurking within the allergic child, and the social behavior of allergic children within the society of children at large.

When she first started working with these groups, Sally would ask who had a Food Allergy Action Plan and medication, and all would raise their hands. However, when she would ask who had their plans and meds with them, they all admitted that their mothers—who were in workshops nearby—were carrying these things for them. Now they all keep these things in their possession at all times.

This is good news from the point of view that the teenagers are taking responsibility for themselves. However, it carries a caution. Sally says that these teenagers are just as daring as their nonallergic counterparts. They feel that because they can carry their medication and action plans with them, they can also go along with their allergy-free friends and partake of most of the same freedoms. If anything goes wrong, they have their rescue medication.

The problem is that the more they take chances, the more can go wrong. Just as the percentages are against teenagers when they drive, they are against teenagers when they push the limits of their medication regimen.

Comfort at Being Among "Your Own Kind"

Those workshops reveal some peer-group concerns that would never occur to us in our clinical practice. For example, there's the matter of food allergy and fashion.

Huh? What do allergies have to do with a teenager's wardrobe?

That's what we say, too. But it's important to boys that they find a place to carry their medication without looking like nerds. Traditionally only dorks and nerds carried pens, combs, and so forth in their shirt pockets. To that add the injectable epinephrine. Girls have purses, so they don't have this problem.

Thus, in one of Ms. Noone's sessions, she was introduced to the phenomenon of "cargo pants," a style that was unfamiliar to her on any practical level—and to us—but that have ample pocket space for hiding an EpiPen from one's nonallergic friends. What we'd like to know is what is going to happen when the style shifts from baggy pants to the skin-tight kind that were popular years ago. "Is that an EpiPen in your pocket or are you just glad to see me?"

Regardless of the particular style, this is the kind of problem young people solve among their peers, and that their parents or we doctors don't have the time or imagination to even think of. These support groups give them an opportunity to swap information they can't get from their nonallergic friends. Kids without these problems can't understand the preoccupation of those who do have them. How can a kid even admit that he's worried about such things, let alone ask for answers?

Fashion, of course, is just one of the myriad problems that get discussed in such groups. How to prepare for travel, or go away to camp or college—these are issues that are solved best by those who face them personally.

The Allergist's Waiting Room: The First Support Group

The precursor of the support group was the allergist's office, which we see as a place of refuge for children who need routine treatment and their parents. This phenomenon has two elements.

One is that children know what to expect when they get there. It might be a shot or a food or other test, but the child knows the limits after a short time.

A trip to the pediatrician, by contrast, is always a surprise for the child. Who knows what will happen when she gets there? It may just be a tongue depressor and an otoscope, which are intrusive enough. But it may also involve a shot, or blood tests, or a probing of parts of the body that no one should ever touch by a child's reckoning—feelings that many adults have never gotten over themselves. Moreover, the diagnosis and treatment will always be a mystery. Will it mean icky medicine? Yuck! Will it mean a shot? Ouch! Will it mean no school, lots of bed rest, and daytime television? Hurray! Will it mean hospitalization? Mommy! And what about all those "other" kids? Who knows what I'll catch from them? Don't leave me!!!

So the trips to the allergist, which always fall within certain limits, may be mildly painful, or even boring, but become reassuring when they become part of an effective routine.

The second element of the allergist's office as refuge is the society of the waiting room. People are tribal. They draw strength from their own kind. And the allergist's waiting room is the first place on earth that parents and children are among their own. The kids gravitate towards each other. They exchange ideas and stories informally. Newcomers are especially delighted to meet someone whose own condition is like their own. Having been made to feel different, even freakish, at school, suddenly they are not alone.

The same is true for parents. In fact, it was waiting room society that inspired our first parents' group many years ago when we watched the veteran mothers give the newcomers ideas about how to cope.

At our office we even go to the extent of holding annual parties for this funny little community that are catered by the patients and parents themselves. Each dish is brought in with the ingredients labeled so that people understand each other's food allergies. Children are delighted when they meet another with the same sensitivity. It gives them a lot to talk about and can lead to play dates and lasting friendship. "At last, a friend I can visit who doesn't have peanut butter in his house! He won't give me a hard time or laugh because I can't even have the peanut butter near me!"

Retention of Information

One of the best things about waiting room society is that it reinforces new information.

Studies show that parents only retain 10 percent of what they hear the first time they hear it. If nothing else, they are often too nervous about their child's condition to take in all that new information. That's why we supplement what we tell them in the office with pamphlets and other reading matter. But we also distribute this material in small doses because we know that they won't read a big stack of new stuff in one sitting. The more we give them, the more likely it is to pile up in the home unread, gathering dust—and we don't want any more dust in their homes. Thus, the professionals are bound to a program of constant reiteration and supplementation during visits, and of course, visits cost money.

The Internet is a useful tool and more and more information is online, although some of it is misleading and even dangerous.

Regardless, there's no substitute for mom-to-mom. When two moms start talking about their kids, the retention rate goes way up. The more experienced mom is a guru, a pathfinder, a sage. The newcomer mom is the wide-eyed student. She listens and takes notes, and they exchange phone numbers. The old-hand mom puts the information exactly in the terms that the newcomer finds most helpful, the voice of experience. She has listened to all that medical talk and recast it in the practical language of "Momhood."

However, the same vulnerabilities that make waiting room culture so effective also leave anxious parents open to quack support groups and treatments, especially online. In our waiting rooms, newcomers learn from our allergy community. They reflect the ideas that we use in our treatment. Thus, they are fairly insulated from screwball ideas and from parents on a misguided, misinformed mission.

College: The Next Watershed Event

College is the time when the child's ability to cope with the world is put to the test. It's not full independence, but it comes close enough. The child goes from a world of curfews and occasional all-nighters eating God knows what to months with little parental oversight. The amount of envelope pushing that goes with a driver's license is squared. College-age kids do their own things for their own reasons.

An asthmatic athlete will ignore his treatment because he thinks it doesn't look tough enough to have a rescue inhaler on the sidelines during practice, or worse, he won't tell the athletic director about his condition, for fear that he won't be allowed to play.

This is just foolish. And potentially catastrophic. But other times, the change offers the opportunity for a sensible re-examination of the whole course of treatment.

For example, a teenager who admits to "cheating" on her food allergy regimen will claim there have been no ill effects. This may be the time to do a food challenge to find out whether the sensitivity is still present or whether the child has become tolerant.

For those on allergy shots, it becomes an opportunity to assess whether there's any need to continue or not. It might be that the allergy shots have worked after two years and, while another year might be a good precaution, there may be sensible reasons to end them early based on the patient's particulars.

A kid who's going to a school like Columbia in New York City, for example, can walk from his dormitory to the infirmary for his shot in a few minutes. However, at the University of Wisconsin or Ohio State, that trip might take half an hour or more. For such a student, once-a-month allergy shots may be too much. So after much discussion and perhaps some skin tests or RAST tests or a food challenge, we may let the immunotherapy slide and pack him off to school with a good supply of oral medications.

Tattoos

As fathers and as physicians, we have noted the fad of tattooing with skeptical eyes. If your children have allergies, you have a new argument against it—if you are given a say in the matter. A study in the *New England Journal of Medicine* (July 2, 2009) documented cases of intense itching of a tattooed area that doesn't respond to topical and intralesional steroids or laser therapy, and necessitates skin excision and grafts. It observed that "hypersensitivity to red pigments is most common, especially those containing mercuric sulfide (cinnabar)."

SEX: THE LAST FRONTIER

This is a particularly troubling issue for all parents. Sex has been the subject of a good deal of propaganda for more than a generation. It has by turns been extolled as liberating and natural on one side and placed on a pedestal (and therefore to be saved for marriage) on the other. The potential medical consequences are well known, as are the protocols limiting transmission of disease. Then there's the old-fashioned problem of pregnancy. As if all the medical considerations weren't enough, sex defines huge fault lines in American politics as well.

What does this have to do with allergy? If you're a young woman—and perhaps a young man—who has a severe peanut allergy, it has a great deal to do with it.

A young female patient of mine arrived in my office one morning with her boyfriend in tow.

She asked me, "Doctor, can I get an anaphylactic reaction from sex?"

I didn't answer right away—part of being a good allergist, after all, is being a good listener, but in this case I was both speechless and wanted to hear more.

The boyfriend said, "She told me about her peanut allergy, and I had some peanuts yesterday so I brushed my teeth and rinsed my mouth out before we went out. We had some wine and went back to her room and one thing led to another ... Suddenly she starts heaving and shaking. I thought I had suddenly turned into the world's greatest lover. So I started going at it even harder, and she starts pounding me on my back. Finally, she pushes me off and grabs her EpiPen and gives herself an injection."

The girl said, "Let me ask again. Can I get anaphylaxis from sex?"

Obviously, that question carries its own answer. I must say this was a new one to me. Let's just say that those allergenic proteins in peanuts are tiny, and just because they are called a "food" allergy doesn't mean they have to be eaten in their traditional form to cause an exposure.

So to the parents of food-allergic children who are "exploring" their sexuality, all I can say is that "safe sex" has a new and important meaning.

— *Dr. Ehrlich*

CHAPTER 14

Mom and the Rest of the Family

MR. MOM

I had a patient, a 4-year-old boy, who was extremely allergic to bananas, probably sensitized at a very young age by spoon-feeding from those little jars you see in every house when solid food is introduced into a baby's diet. His mother was very conscientious about keeping bananas out of the home. She read labels scrupulously and warned people not to feed him bananas in any form. In fact, her care bordered on the obsessive in the eyes of her husband and her mother-in-law. After all, weren't bananas good for you? Weren't they "natural" snacks? Some people thought that bananas were making Mom bananas herself.

Then one Sunday while her husband and child were visiting her in-laws and she was enjoying a morning off with the newspaper, she got a call from her anxious, and very contrite, husband from the emergency room. He had fed the boy a piece of his own mother's specialty—banana cream pie. "I thought, 'it's not really bananas,'" he explained later. The child survived anaphylaxis, and from then on, Dad was a very zealous convert to the cause of keeping bananas away from his son.

— *Dr. Ehrlich*

THE ONLY THING SURPRISING ABOUT STORIES LIKE THIS IS THAT there are so many of them. Why do people continue to believe that they somehow know better than the doctor or the attentive mother? Why do so many children end up in emergency rooms? You would think that when a child is diagnosed with a specific medical condition, everyone close to him or her would bend over backwards to help keep to the regimen. But while allergies can be life-threatening, there's something about them that breeds skepticism, conscious or unconscious.

Allergies set in motion a difficult set of dynamics in most families. The more serious the allergies are, the more they tend to upset the family equilibrium. Like other chronic illnesses, such as alcoholism or diabetes, allergies elicit complicated emotions, with a desire to protect the ill child on the one hand and jealousy over the attention from the primary caregiver(s) on the other. Included is some combination of shame about the genetics of allergy and shame over past and current behavior. The illness is both a fact of life and, on some level, a deep, dark secret to be kept. One of the difficulties families have in coping with allergies is facing up not only to the physical disease in their midst but the subtle distorting effects they have on the rest of the family. Allergies expose or exacerbate subtle psychological and cultural differences between parents, and particularly between spouses and their in-laws.

These issues need to be addressed. Otherwise, allergy can rob family life of its joy, and childhood of its innocence and excitement, both for the allergic child and nonallergic siblings.

THE HELPING HAND

Those of you who were addicted to *The Sopranos* for its many-year run on HBO may recall that Tony is able to trace his propensity for black outs and anxiety attacks to earlier generations of his family. Based on custom and a sense of shame, however, these events were glossed over and called by other names. In the earlier mob movie *Mean Streets*, a girl with epilepsy is referred to as "sick in the head." (The director, Martin Scorsese, couldn't take part in many activities as a child because he had severe asthma.)

Italians are hardly the only ethnic group that harbors a sense of embarrassment over chronic illness, as Dr. Ehrlich shows elsewhere in this book. Among old-time Italians, however, such conditions are seen as the result of the "evil eye." A case of asthma is hidden from the community because it is evidence of guilt and punishment for some evil someone in the family has done, and the culture stresses the importance of family responsibility over individual actions.

They also have a folk saying: "Your children should be like the fingers of your hand; you do not love one finger more than the other."

As an American allergist of Italian descent, I would like to see the superstition of the first idea supplanted by the enlightenment of the second.

— *Dr. Chiaramonte*

What happens when you hit a finger with a hammer? Your whole hand is affected. Your grip gets weaker. The other fingers must compensate for the injury or the hand becomes dysfunctional.

When your child has bad allergies or asthma, strange things happen. You do not love the sick child more than the others, but he commands more of your attention. Having an asthmatic or allergic child changes the dynamics of your family, just as having a dislocated or broken finger will change the way you use the whole hand.

Chronic illnesses like asthma, diabetes, and alcoholism affect the whole family. As family members try to compensate for the illness of one kid, they become codependent with the "identified ill child." It seems as if the family members need the "identified ill person" not to get better to keep balance in the family. As the parents rally to the support of the ill child, other children can lose out. It might almost be better if everyone were ill.

Ideally, other members of the family should rise to the challenge and selflessly support the afflicted. But we would also like to see the ill child become as normal a part of customary family life as is possible. Their special medical needs should not set them apart. Instead, they should be integrated into the lives of the others *before* the illness upsets the delicate balance that any family constitutes in these challenging times. No one should become the "forgotten" child or even, as often happens, the "forgotten" spouse.

But first things first. While we don't want to see any family's happiness compromised by allergies, each family must first develop the knowledge and discipline necessary to keep the condition itself under control. This is a battle, and every battle requires a commander in the field.

The Designated-Parent Theory

In two-parent families, one parent inevitably emerges as the primary caregiver.

This parent's job is to learn everything practical about the condition, and the learning curve is steep. This would involve attending allergist appointments with the child, reading the literature, learning how to administer medication, and seeing that it gets done. Further duties are shopping for the child, seeing that conditions in the home meet the recommended guidelines, and seeing that the child travels with whatever level of "protective bubble" is necessary to preclude an event during the time she is away from home.

It's not that two parents can't become equally authoritative, but it's hard work, and this initial job of acquiring expertise will absorb a disproportionate amount of a parent's time. Someone has to attend to other parts of the family's lives during this first, intensive phase of adjustment. Two parents focused equally on allergies and asthma can mean equal neglect of other children and the marriage itself.

Moreover, the child needs a coherent authority, one voice he or she can go to get the straight story. The other adults in the process should have the information funneled through the same channel. If the other

---

THE DECIDERS

I make it a rule that in a two-parent situation, the family and I decide who will be the primary parent. This approach is very important with respect to food allergies because the possibility of giving the child mixed messages may have dire consequences.

I am reminded of an 8-year-old child who was allergic to peanuts and whose father bought him some candy. Mother had spoken of cross-contamination of foods, and all were aware of what might happen if there was ingestion of food with peanuts in it. Father bought a cookie for his child one day at a bakery when they were out taking a walk. He asked the bakery employees if the cookie contained peanuts and if there might be contamination. "No" and "no." His son bit into the cookie and had a mild reaction. Sonny Boy squealed to mother saying that he had had a reaction to a cookie bought at The Village Bakery.

"What!?" screamed mother. "*Everybody* knows not to buy cookies there because they are all baked on the same cookie sheets!"

The implication of Mom's choice of words, of course, is that *everybody* does not include Dad.

Moral: Better to be safe than sorry. Let *one* parent be entirely responsible for what and where to eat.   — *Dr. Chiaramonte*

spouse or the grandparents become avid participants in the process, there can be splintering and distortion of the message that will result in misleading, possibly contradictory directions for the child, potentially ending in the emergency room. The designated parent will be the one who has been to the doctor's office, sat in the support groups, read the newsletters, and so on. She will also be the one who has seen the effects of the allergen, not just learned the cause. In the anecdote that started the chapter, the key word for Mom was "banana"; for Dad and Grandma it was "pie." Dad got religion only after his kid almost died. In the cookie anecdote, the key word was "peanuts" not "minute peanut residue." The emotional subtext was "Let's have a little fun while we're out of the house," not "We have to be careful because 'Big Mother' is watching."

This single-authority model is a difficult concept for parents to assimilate at times. It is contrary to the idea of cooperative, complementary, involved parenting that is now the norm. In most cases, two active parents balance each other. There's nothing wrong in most cases where the child has to make sense out of the differences between the two parents. It's one thing when Dad likes action movies, while Mom thinks they're too violent. Or Dad may want Sonny to stand up to bullies at school, where Mom wants to transfer him out. But where the school-of-hard-knocks theory does teach a child to get on in the world in many cases, with allergies the results can be disastrous.

YOU CAN'T TRUST THE GRANDPARENTS

There are times when an "expert" becomes just another thoughtless, doting grandparent. I got a call one weekend from an angry Mom, whose daughter had reacted to a piece of orange given to her by Grandpa. Fortunately, this was not a life-threatening event, but it was nasty enough, made worse for Grandpa by the mother's fury. She was right. Grandpa should have known better!
The little girl was my own granddaughter.   — *Dr. Ehrlich*

The ideal is not to fuss over allergic children every minute of the day, but to make them their own monitors. Of course this is related to the child's level of maturity. During infancy and early childhood, parental protection is required. Adolescent rebellion must exclude taking chances with allergy treatment. Anaphylactic shock is not like getting a bloody nose or even throwing up because you sneak liquor from the old man's liquor cabinet. Out in the world, a child must be able to say "I can't eat that" even if he risks being seen as a finicky eater or a killjoy. We know one extended family of good cooks who go crazy because the child travels with his own supply of hot dogs and macaroni and cheese. They know better than to feed him anything with peanuts, but the child's fear of new food has narrowed his tastes. Those are the breaks. Better a picky eater than an evening at the hospital.

The child must be able to resist the mistakes of friends and friends' parents. He must also be able to say no to Grandma who might tell him, "A little won't hurt you." The fact is that "a little" taste of the offending substance *will* deliver it into allergen central for distribution to all key body parts. The body's defenses will order in airborne troops and carpet-bombing. Shoot first and ask questions later.

When the child is an infant and toddler, you do have a big say in his or her daily activities and eating habits. Controlling these environments are a necessity because the child lacks an understanding of the importance of avoiding allergens—and the consequences if he or she does not.

But the process of shifting responsibility can begin fairly young. By the age of 3 or 4, most children become very savvy about their allergies because they know how bad they feel if they are exposed to an offending allergen. Many children will alert a parent when there is imminent danger.

Now Batting for the Allergic Child: Mom

You will notice that in these anecdotes Mom is the authority and Dad is the fool. We have nothing against dads; we both are dads. We have used he or she randomly to refer to a single child just because it's awkward to use the plural they and related grammatical constructions all the time and we don't want to look sexist. But in the case of the designated parent, there is a tinge of gender bias based entirely on our clinical experience. Designated parents are generally moms.

everal years ago one of my very sweet 4-year-old patients, who happened to be severely milk allergic, went out for a walk in Greenwich Village with his father on a Sunday morning. As they passed a stationery store the boy begged his father to buy him a candy bar. After checking a label on one for the word "milk" and finding none, the father paid for the candy and handed it to his son. He watched his son looking at the label without removing it from the wrapper as they walked on University Place. After a few minutes, his son suddenly said, "Daddy, what does 'casein' mean?"

His father grabbed the item, and, sure enough, the last ingredient on the label was the milk protein casein. His son had recognized potential disaster. Not because he understood what casein meant, but because he had been taught to question anything out of the ordinary; disaster was averted. Mom went to bed that night proud of her son instead of mad at Dad.

— *Dr. Ehrlich*

Dads tend to be skeptical of allergies, especially when their sons are afflicted. "Allergies are for *wusses* ... They're a sign of weakness ... Life is full of small indignities—he'll never grow up if he has to read labels all the time ... Besides, his mother drives me crazy with her constant talk about it ... We can't go out to dinner without giving the third degree to a waiter." These are common attitudes among dads. To make things worse, dads are worried that their kids won't be able to become amateur athletes, let alone professional superstars.

Grandparents can be worse, especially if the tendency towards allergy comes from their son-in-law's or daughter-in-law's line. "*We* don't have allergies ... *They* are neurotic ... *They* are weak ... *She/He* never shuts up ... *She/He* tries to run our house when they come over—*we* can't change the way we live because *she/he* has a problem ... What's childhood without chocolate/bananas/peanut butter/the dog/you name it?"

Childhood is supposed to be a time of boundless possibilities. It's a time when people say to their children, "Work hard and there's nothing you can't do." But the parents of children with allergies are in the position of saying, "Work hard and there's nothing you can't do, except have a dog or eat peanuts or sleep in the woods at camp.

There's nothing you can't do as long as you carry your medicine, take it faithfully, and remain within a three-mile radius of an emergency room."

Enforcing these rules is a tough job but someone's gotta do it, and the best enforcers, besides the children themselves when they are old and mature enough (we hope), are their mothers.

Not that dads can't do it, but as a rule, moms take a disproportionate share of responsibility for the child's well-being anyway. Even at schools where there's a heavy quotient of parental involvement, mothers attend parent-teacher conferences without their husbands at least half the time, according to one principal we know, and the number of times husbands go without their wives is no more than ten percent. Moms go to the doctor with the child, shop for the family groceries and children's clothes, and are generally more fastidious about the child's routine. They are the ones who read the parenting magazines and parenting books and talk with their friends about parenting issues.

Certainly if there is role reversal on these issues, the opposite can be done. If, for example, the father is the stay-at-home parent and the mother works out of the house.

Or if the grandparents or nannies take a custodial part in the child's life because both parents work, they can do some of it too. But by and large, given the apportioning of household responsibility in two-parent families or custody in one-parent families, Mom is it.

Having said this, we must also raise questions about how far to go. While selfless devotion is desirable and necessary at the start of the process, we must also sound cautionary alarms about carrying it to extremes.

CODEPENDENCE—NOW WHO'S THE SICK ONE?

Mrs. Jones's baby had a severe allergic reaction to cow's milk in infancy. She spent the next fourteen years having her son avoid cow's milk, reading labels, and having EpiPen available just in case. Her husband felt overlooked for this and other reasons. They separated. *(continued on next page)*

One Saturday, she called our emergency service and told the operator with alarm that her milk-allergic son had eaten ice cream at a birthday party. We called back and asked her what his symptoms were. She said, "Nothing!"

So we told her to keep an eye on him and if anything happened one of us would meet her at the emergency room, but if he showed no symptoms she should bring him in on Monday.

Monday morning arrived—a school day—and there they were when the office opened. We asked the mother to sit in the reception room and questioned the boy about when he had started eating ice cream. "A few months ago." Any problems? "No. I told my mother but she did not believe me. My father just said good and that my mother was a worrywart." Any other milk products? "Chocolate milk."

So I asked Mom to return and told her that the boy appeared to have outgrown—for now—his problem with milk. That it was not uncommon with some food allergies—peanuts being a notable exception. She was so skeptical that we administered a series of low-tech tests. Milk on the skin. Milk on the lips. Ingestion of small amounts of milk, gradually increasing to, finally, a whole glass.

Instead of joy, the mother fainted. She recovered and sat there in disbelief. She finally turned to me and said, "What will I do now?"

— *Dr. Ehrlich*

Mrs. Jones's story is a prime example of an unintended consequence of good, hands-on, preventive allergy care. Namely, that parents and patients alike will find ways to use the fact of the illness to unhealthy advantage.

Patients will find ways to use the illness to manipulate the behavior of the people around them. A child—for example, an adolescent asthmatic boy who doesn't like undressing in the locker room for physical education—might tell Mom to write him a note saying he is feeling wheezy that day and can he please be excused from gym? Or a girl who thinks that after a shower she will be unable to put on makeup and look her best will do the same thing.

With the Mrs. Joneses of the world, the problem is that they invest so much of themselves in the child's illness that it becomes an intrinsic part of their identity. Mrs. Jones spent all her psychic and physical energy protecting her child and in the process neglected other dimensions of her life; her husband became her ex-husband. The consensus of all her friends is that "She's a saint." Who needs more affirmation than that? But as anyone who has read *Saint Joan* by George Bernard Shaw can attest, saints can have problems in their dealings with mere mortals.

Addressing these dynamics is the purview of family therapy, as we have touched on earlier. The field of family therapy departs from traditional therapy by focusing on the family and the complex interactions among its members instead of the individual. However, we must recognize that it's not something that every family can or will avail itself of, or will only avail itself of when it has already begun to suffer as a group.

Some fifty to sixty years ago, Dr. Murray Pushpin at Mount Sinai Hospital in New York City and later at Denver's Children's Asthma Hospital observed a telling phenomenon. When hospitalized under optimal conditions, some children improved quickly—what are called "rapid remitters"—only to start wheezing and coughing the minute Mom came to visit. Another study showed that some patients remitted rapidly when the parents took a vacation and the kids stayed at home, supervised by medical personnel. Pushpin coined the word "parentectomy" to describe this inverse link between the child's health and the parent's presence.

We now recognize that families are complex in their relationships. In a family, the "patient" is not the only one who is affected by the illness. Each member of the family plays a role, although the patient is the "star." Thus the basis for the field of family therapy, in which the entire family is treated. Today, with the multiple models for the family unit, a more apt term might be household therapy.

The central theme is that without therapy, other family members function as enablers. By helping the ill person deal with the chronic illness, the others eventually come to define their existence and derive purpose in life from their supporting roles to the patient-star. This is the nature of that well-known phenomenon, codependency.

It took us doctors a long time to learn this. We are trained to look at individuals. However, when institutions are involved—with residential treatment for alcoholics and asthmatics alike—the perspectives of other trained observers come into play. Social workers. Psychologists. They have provided the larger perspective that MDs lacked, and, in the case of much allergy and asthma treatment today, the larger perspective that many overworked MDs still don't have.

Some of the seminal work in this field was done, of course, by the affected populations themselves. The alcoholics at AA began to learn about these relationships and provided their insights to social workers, who then became specialists in family dynamics. They did family-tree studies going back generations of alcohol addiction and the way others adapted to it. They found the skeletons in family closets and traced their effects on family attitudes.

It may hurt to hear that a condition like life-threatening asthma or food allergy can be mentioned in the same breath as alcoholism, but it is necessary. To the extent that stress is a factor in treatment (See chapter 10, "Alternative Treatments"), family dynamics are critical.

Our practices were instrumental in founding some of the first parent support groups for asthma and food allergy in the country, and we strongly recommend the idea to those who are just beginning to come to grips with the kind of treatment that we espouse here. Just as alcoholics and the families of alcoholics often possess the best insights into the personal and family dynamics of their affliction, so parental and peer affinity groups are often true experts on asthma and food allergy. They are sympathetic to newcomers. And in a field where so much law and regulation is still evolving along with the medicine, they are the best researchers. We learn from them all the time.

Nothing gives us greater satisfaction than sitting back and having our support-group veterans take new members through their paces. They have been there and they have the knack of explaining not only the *whats*, *wheres*, and *hows* to newcomers in jargon-free language, but the *whys* as well. They are particularly good at tempering the zeal of new converts into constructive incremental thinking.

Quack, Quack!

We also recommend that you align yourselves with support groups that have good professional guidance—an allergist or someone else with credentials that are rooted in the kind of treat ment we talk about in this book. No amateurs or Dr. Feelgoods.

The nature of allergic disease makes it fertile ground for quacks, who promise cures using brown rice and herbs, or who demonize factors that are outside the realm of medical science. A reader review of the earlier incarnation of this book complained precisely that it didn't offer some natural panacea, but that's not the way we work.

The title MD is no guarantee of integrity. There are doctors who will test and treat allergy under any code they can bill for. They are to be avoided. There are patients who think that anything they get off the Internet must be more reliable than anything their doctor tells them. The American Academy of Allergy, Asthma & Immunology has position statements (online at www.aaaai.org) on what most good allergists think about different types of treatment.

For families that are facing years of disciplined treatment, there's nothing more attractive than the idea of a quick cure, but don't hold your breath (no pun intended) waiting for one to come along. The ideal support group will be one that helps you get through the hardest parts with your judgment intact. It will be informative and earnest without being fanatical. It will project the message, "Been there, done that," and explain how you and your family can do it too.

Good humor and some detachment are necessities, individually and collectively. The last thing we want for the mothers of our newly milk-tolerant patients is to answer the question, "What do I do now?" with the words, "I'll start a support group." At least not without a long vacation, a couple of graduate courses, and perhaps a new shade of lipstick or a new wardrobe first.

GETTING STARTED ON YOUR SUPPORT GROUP

Kathy Lundquist, a member of FAAN's Advisory Council, gave these tips for planning support group meetings, with certain small additions by the authors. They are for food allergy, but could easily be adapted for asthma and other conditions:

• Plan topics for each meeting, including milk-free recipes, shopping tips, scouting safe restaurants, or educating PTAs, preschools, and church groups. *(continued on next page)*

• Arrange for guest speakers (and guest listeners) including pediatricians, allergists, nurses, dermatologists, dieticians, model school representatives, psychologists, and others who are in a position to either supply information or who have a lot to learn.
• Have a specific agenda and begin and end on time.
• Divide responsibility. People will support the things they help create. Try to involve passive members in organizational activities and they will become more involved.
• Have a co-leader to help take some of the burden off the leader.

The Rest of the Family

We certainly would not pretend to be experts at family therapy. Nonetheless, we would like to point to certain factors within our purview as allergists that you might find helpful as you seek to cope with the medical issues. In our field, we do see common challenges to families with allergic children whose illnesses demand life style changes from others. We will suggest some ways of dealing with these changes. Each family is different so there is no one best way of doing this, but the broad outlines are fairly clear.

In general, we would like to see our patients' families look at the affirmative possibilities in their situation. As we say elsewhere in the book: When life hands you a lemon, make lemonade.

ALLERGY SHOULDN'T BE A DARK FAMILY SECRET

One of the joys of practicing in New York City is that it is, in the words of a former mayor, not a melting pot but "a gorgeous mosaic" of cultures and ethnicities from all over the globe. This gives a doctor a window on many worlds.

But not all our insights are heartwarming. We had an asthmatic teenage girl from a close-knit ethnic enclave—I won't mention which one—in one of the boroughs outside Manhattan. Her progress under our treatment was so remarkable that her excited father showed up at a parents' support group we run in Manhattan. Dad was so impressed that he *(continued on next page)*

---

decided he would like to start such a group in his own neighborhood because the benefits could then be brought to his own people
without their having to venture into an alien world.

I thought, "This is real progress. To be able to reach into an insular
community where asthma is very common with the energy of a
modern support group." But my excitement lasted about eighteen
hours. The phone rang at the office. "My husband means well," said
the woman's accented voice on the phone, "but he is a fool. He can't
start such a group in our community."

"Why not?" I asked. "You have seen the good it has done for your
daughter, and I'm sure there are others who could benefit in your
neighborhood."

"What you say is true, doctor," she said, "and believe me I am very
grateful for the change you have made in our child's quality of life.
But, you must understand that if we let the rest of the community
know that she is sick, she will never find a husband." — *Dr. Ehrlich*

While this may be a story about life outside what some might
call the mainstream of American life, it does reflect a tendency that
extends far beyond the confines of a largely self-contained ethnic
community. That is, to think that the allergic child is blighted and
there is something shameful about her illness. No matter how modern
or enlightened, people tend to curse their genes, curse their prenatal
diet, curse their pets, and now with the "pound-of-dirt theory" that
says we are too clean and too hygienic, who knows? They'll probably
curse their housekeeping.

While some would hide the illness because it interferes with a
ritual view of marriageability, at the other end of the spectrum are
those who expect the rest of the world to bend to them. The parents
are so aggressive in trying to make the world safe for their allergic
children that they are probably neglecting the emotional needs of
the rest of the family, including themselves, and alienating the larger
community.

As far as we are concerned, the two points of view—hiding the
illness and brandishing it like a battle flag—are closer than you might
imagine, and neither is satisfactory. Allergy is not a condition that

should be hidden from the light of day, but neither should it be waved around like a cross in a world of vampires.

Anne Muñoz-Furlong, founder of the Food Allergy & Anaphylaxis Network, was asked if she would support a ban on peanut butter in schools. Her answer was, "It's not a peanut butter–less world." Her reasoning is that you can't change the world to fit the needs of the few. Rather, you equip the few with the tools they need to make their way, nurturing the child from dependence to independence.

A Dog's Life

A new element has entered the peanut allergy discussion since we wrote the first edition of this book, which is the training of dogs to detect peanuts in the child's vicinity. Inspired by drug- and bomb-sniffing dogs, these animals travel with their kids to malls and birthday parties—anywhere they might encounter stray allergens. The pooches carry emergency medication in special pouches.

We feel that children with sensitivity levels so extreme that they might benefit—down to fleeting exposure to dust or touch, as opposed to actual ingestion—are rare. The economics are extreme: $10,000 to $15,000 to train each dog, so it's hardly a mass solution. Carrying injectable rescue medication—EpiPen or Twinject—is an effective fail-safe. Dr. Sampson's research shows that fatalities generally result from unexpected exposure, like climbing a mountain with a companion who is carrying energy bars that contain trace peanuts. Or when someone who is unaware of their allergy is exposed to peanuts a second time. Under any other circumstances, a 911 call should bring life-saving relief in time.

Finally, traveling with Fido could engender a false sense of security, and somehow excuse parent and child from developing the skills they need to be vigilant on their own behalf. You can't take a dog with you everywhere. Does that mean a child can only go where his "bubble" will allow?

And we can envision the day when the peanut-allergic kids face off against the dog-allergic ones. Something's got to give.

Allergic children, even severely allergic children, don't need the message that the world has been unfair to them and that it can always be made to conform to their needs. Allergic and asthmatic children have rights under the law, including the Americans with Disabilities Act (ADA). This is an admirable law. But its spirit is not always well served by constantly pushing it to the limits. People in wheelchairs have a right to conduct their lives as normally as possible, but should the ADA be used to force a school district to pay for an assistant so that a teacher with severe dyslexia can teach English, as was the case in one upstate New York town? Do we want our children to think of themselves as handicapped, or perhaps, in contemporary jargon, "immunologically challenged"?

We don't believe so. We believe that families should try to work with their special challenges to make their lives special. Robert Frost was once asked if he didn't think it would be liberating to ignore traditional formal poetic constraints like rhyme and meter, as was then in vogue, to just let his imagination go. His reply, "Tennis with the net down is fun, but it's not so good a game."

Allergy and asthma are not a game. They are frequently a matter of life and death. But that doesn't mean that life itself shouldn't be lived. Families where a member is chronically ill are often suffused with gloom, resentment, and paranoia. Not a good constructive atmosphere.

We ask that all our patients' families try to live life to its fullest, given the special constraints and responsibilities of the illness. This is not easy to do. It is possible to unconsciously consign all of life to the back burner while taking care of a child. But if the possibility is understood from the beginning, it is possible to forge a family life that is every bit as rewarding, and perhaps even closer, than those of "normal" families.

Never sell short your children's capacity to cope with the complexities of the situation. Use some imagination in trying to convey the arcana of allergy. Just as we have resorted to comparisons to Sherlock Holmes and military metaphors to get across the sense of storytelling structure that we find in our work, you can turn the allergic mechanism into an extension of the fairy tales that you read to your children.

We have one acquaintance who, in trying to get across the idea of how the immune system that once fought parasites has emerged thousands of years later to hurt us, compared it to the mummy in the movies. "The mummy was a good guy, but he was locked in a tomb for thousands of years, and when he got out, he was mad at the world and wanted to get even. But don't worry—just like in the movies, the good guys are going to win. And we're the good guys."

We're not going to say that one approach works for everyone, but it's a worthy try. Maybe you can find some stories of your own.

The Rituals of Food

Meals are traditionally one of the settings in which a whole family can reaffirm that the individuals are a family. Yet, with modern life as pressured as it is, one of the ingredients that is frequently missing at meals is *time*, not *thyme*, although that may be missing, too. The family rituals of dining have been under attack for generations anyway.

Having a child with a food allergy limits one of the options that is there for time-challenged families, namely the ability to casually go out to dinner or order takeout, or for the allergic patient to eat on the fly when others have different plans. Managing diet requires deliberation.

Complicated, isn't it?

SOME IDEAS FOR TURNING FOOD AND MEALTIME INTO POSITIVES FOR THE WHOLE FAMILY

• Teach everyone to read labels—not just the child with allergies. Line up the cans and boxes and go over the ingredients. This will not only help the children with their reading but it will foster a sense of solidarity among family members.

• Take everyone shopping. Armed with their new vocabulary, a shopping trip can be almost like a treasure hunt.

• Cook together. Small children can learn their way around a kitchen starting with simple tasks like tearing up lettuce for salads. There are myriad reasons to justify early cooking lessons—training fine motor skills, teaching process by following recipes, forging habits of greater cooperation, and on and on. But mostly, it can be a lot of fun.

As families are eating fewer meals together, the ones they do share become more important. Yet, if anything, meals at home can pose even greater logistical challenges. Do you cook separately for the allergic child? If so, the afflicted child will be tempted by the forbidden food. Do you cook the same things? If the allergen being avoided is a staple of the "average" family diet like wheat, soy, eggs, milk, or peanut butter, it can be quite difficult on the nonallergic family members. It also depends at what age the family members are started on the low-allergy diet. If it is early enough they might not notice the difference. Children who have such allergies are taught rightly to be wary of unfamiliar foods and food from strangers. But do you convey that wariness to everyone in your family? In general, children are picky-enough eaters. You don't want to convey that sense of pickiness to your nonallergic children.

The dietary strictures are just one aspect of what happens within the family. Emotional walls go up along with the dietary limitations. Foods are not eaten and feelings are left unexpressed. These emotional limitations do real damage.

PINING FOR PIGNOLI

My wife had a deadly allergy to *pignoli*—pine nuts—which are staples of Italian cuisine. We never had pine nuts in our home. Our kids were raised not knowing the joys of *pesto*, a sauce made largely of basil and pine nuts. I felt like a rabbi raising his children without bagels.

Once when the children were substantially grown up, my wife went out of state to see her sick sister, leaving me to play Mr. Mom with our three children. We were sitting in an Italian restaurant when the waiter mentioned a pesto special. They asked what it was. I explained it, and they all tried it. It was as if an Italian had discovered America all over again. The rest of the meal consisted of gorging themselves on this delicacy and revelations from my children about what it was like to have an allergic mother and a father who was an allergist. It was obvious to me that much had been left unsaid about life in general as our family steered our way around Mom's allergies over the years. *Buon Appetito.*

— *Dr. Chiaramonte*

Sibling Medication

Most moderate to severe allergic or asthmatic children need to be supervised to take their medication at least twice daily. That's at least two times a day the parental figure's attention is drawn away from the well children. How do you reduce the feelings of neglect on the part of the well children?

Get them to act as assistant caregivers and help the parent give the medication. When you take the medication down from its *secure* location, give it to your assistant to carry. Secure storage is crucial— you don't want anyone to play doctor when you're not around.

Explain each step as your physician taught it to you. Repeat the names of the medications and delivery devices. Take the mystery out of medication and replace it with fun and understanding.

Reinforce the message—and take the attraction out of all the attention that comes from being sick—by playing a game of role reversal. The sick child can act out becoming the assistant caregiver for the well child.

Above all, make sure that all children get time during which they are your sole focus.

Attitude

Of course, in panic mode, there is no way to make allergy into a game. There's no such thing as equal time for the other children during a severe asthma attack or anaphylactic reaction. What will the atmosphere in the family be—hysteria or a cool, reasoned, deliberate response? Parents set the tone for both the ill child and well children. Panic is contagious; calm is catching. Calm leads to effective management.

The most important thing to remember about allergic emergencies is that they are preventable, so managing the disease is the most important preparation you can make.

However, while emergencies are preventable, they do happen. When they do, the allergic child becomes the sole object of the parents' attention, particularly if there's a trip to the emergency room involved. The parents disappear with the sick child, while the siblings stay with the neighbors, wondering if they're ever going to see brother and sister again, or if the ambulance will crash. This is a time for the imagination to run wild, or if it happens often enough, to say, "Here we go again." Resentment builds. Bad thoughts about the sick child start to intrude. Guilt alternates with anger. At the first opportunity, call the well children to reassure them and inform them of the sick child's status.

Here again, understanding is a key. The well children should understand what is happening to their brother or sister during the emergency and why it is important to let their parents devote such attention. Their innate sense of responsibility can be cultivated. They should be taught that they are an important part of the team. They have the responsibility to hold the fort while the parents go off to the hospital. And above all, they should command quality time in equal measure after the emergency is over.

Sports and Other Activities

The allergic child may have true limits: Running in cold air may bring on wheezing and shortness of breath, for instance. For their part, the well children may take this opportunity to shine, to forge an identity outside the home, with all its special rules. Let them go as far as they want. Teams provide an alternative social structure to the close-knit, regulated home—an important outlet even when there is no allergy in the home, but even more crucial where a sick child is the focal point of so much psychic and physical energy.

As for the allergic child, provide the best allergy care you can and then let them find a level of activity that they are comfortable with. Kids are good at finding their own limits; just let them know these may change at different times depending on their status at the start of activities.

Where There's Smoke, There's Allergy

Of course allergic children should not smoke. How about their parents? Quite apart from the fact that secondhand smoke is a hazard for the health of even nonallergic people and is poison for the allergic, the children's role models should not smoke. When we were growing up, parents smoked routinely. (See the movie *Good Night, and Good Luck* which was set in the 1950s or the cable television show *Mad Men* set in the 1960s for a glimpse of the bad old days of cigarettes.

Naturally, kids back then imitated their parents by stealing their cigarettes and hid them from parents until they could sneak off and light up. Those children are today's addicted smokers, and once again they are hiding their habit only now it's from their own kids. If you must smoke, do so only outside the home.

PETS

This is a tough one. All the bromides about the importance of pets to small children—teaching responsibility, empathy, and so on—are true. Children love pets. Children benefit from pets. But what about an allergic child? The pet-in-the-home research we referred to earlier doesn't mitigate the problems furry animals cause in homes where allergy already exists.

Speaking to parents about having a cat or dog at home because of a child's allergy is an issue in my office several times a week. Often I find that the parent knows the problem and the pediatrician knows the problem, but would rather palm it off on me so that I'll be the bad guy. But sometimes that doesn't even help.

Several years ago a veteran patient came into the office with her fiancé, a confirmed dog owner. He wanted to hear it from me that her allergies were bad, and then told me that he would rearrange his living situation to accommodate her allergies. When her allergies were no better after they married and were living together, she presented him with an ultimatum: It's the dog or me. He presented her with divorce papers *the next day*.

Don't get me started about the family with the boa constrictor!

— *Dr. Ehrlich*

Just some observations from years of practice: It is the allergist's job to give the best advice he or she can—no pets. The patient's job is to be honest—"We need a pet."

To this understandable assertion, the best medical answer may be, "How about goldfish?" Given modern reality, the answer may be a dog with short hair or non-shedding characteristics (like the Obamas' dog) instead of a cat, bathed frequently and made to sleep outside, with allergy shots for the patient. — *Dr. Chiaramonte*

Taking Control of Your Child's Allergies and Asthma

Nature's Dirty Trick

T HE ALLERGIC RESPONSE IS ONE OF NATURE'S DIRTY TRICKS. As we have said repeatedly, it is a perfectly useful immune mechanism. But deprived of its natural prey—the parasites that plagued our ancestors in the cradles of civilization—it comes back to target the wrong things, and so deprive its victims of a normal, comfortable life.

Allergy is just one of several immunity dramas being played out currently as nature fights back against "progress," along with the emergence of HIV and antibiotic-resistant strains of bacteria. All show that there are mechanisms, whether actually "intelligent" or not, that fight hard to survive in the face of assault by science and technology.

The overall fight between medicine and disease is constant, and while medicine has held an advantage since the invention of penicillin, that lead is now threatened. The battle between allergy and medicine, on the other hand, has been very close for a long time, and it is not always clear who is ahead.

One thing we do know, as should be clear after reading this book, is that the allergy battle will never be won by fighting on too narrow a footing. The allergic mechanisms are both immediate and slow acting. Remember the military complexity of allergy, corresponding to paratroops, carpet-bombing, and land mines. They threaten our comfort, our overall health, and even our lives in both the short and long run. We have to be at least as resourceful in fighting them.

Not all our foes are locked inside the mast cells and basophils either. Some of them are economic, some are bureaucratic, and some are behavioral—our own and that of our children.

We are all accustomed to railing against insurance companies as the embodiment of all that is wrong with our medical system. They have earned the scorn of their patients, the companies that pay them,

---

AN ECONOMIC CHOICE, NOT A MEDICAL ONE

Once an HMO offered me the chance to become a consultant, and asked for a proposal for guidelines on how many lung-function tests they should pay for per year for asthmatics. This was a false proposition because the effectiveness of treatment varies from patient to patient. It was obvious what they wanted: someone who would set aggressive guidelines, i.e., a low number, that would minimize their costs.

Also in the competition for this contract was a former student of mine who low-balled his proposal—deliberately setting a low number—and won the contract. Medicine is a business as well as a healing art, especially in this day and age. Some of us are more business oriented than others. *— Dr. Chiaramonte*

---

and the doctors who belong to them. You will have to wait a long time to hear either one of us say anything in their defense.

The problem with the health care system is that no one wants to pay for it. Taxpayers don't want to pick up the tab for universal health care, which would be a more profound reform than simply universal insurance. The companies that contract with health-insurance companies want to lower their costs and try to put the squeeze on the insurance companies, although the insurance companies seem to routinely raise their premiums by double digits every year while requiring the insured to bear more and more of their costs. Workers don't want to lose more of their take-home pay. Stockholders, including many of us through our pensions and mutual funds, don't want to see insurance companies lose more of their market value by being too good to patients. Doctors, including your authors, don't want to work *pro bono*. And on and on.

All any of these groups are doing is shifting their costs to other links in this daisy chain. It's often a better business practice for an insurance company to "just say no" to treatment, than it is to say yes. Why? They may be prepared to pay the bill in the end, but it's also possible that they will escape some of their obligations simply because patients and doctors won't have the stamina to keep on arguing. Or, God forbid, the patient may die. In the meantime, the insurance companies have achieved greater productivity by shifting administrative costs onto their patients or network doctors, who pay for HMO efficiency by becoming less efficient themselves.

Don't get us started!

Of course, this cost shifting is like a bubble in a carpet. The bubble doesn't go away when you step on it, it merely resurfaces elsewhere. The economic costs multiply as cheaper disease management under the care of specialists is transmuted into emergency treatment and hospitalization—higher costs that are eventually borne by everyone.

The tragedy is that the bubble carries not merely an economic cost, but a cost in quality of life and the patient's long-term health. Sleepless nights, school absences, curtailed physical activity, losing out on the normal joy of childhood experience, permanently diminished lung capacity—those are costs you can't shift.

Partners in Treatment

In our first chapter, we spoke of allergic children, parents, and GPs, pediatricians, and allergists all being partners in treating allergy. To this list we should add another partner—your child's body—because sometimes it seems to have a mind of its own, and sometimes, if properly trained, it can do a better job of treating your child than the rest of us can. That's part of the message of our chapters on immunotherapy and the environment. Because the mechanisms of allergy have survived millennia of "progress," we have a good deal to gain by trying to use the body's own resources to reduce its capacity to attack itself, or to remove, as much as possible, its excuses for doing so.

Someone who has thought this through very clearly, and has written and spoken on the subject quite eloquently, is Nancy Sander of Allergy & Asthma Network Mothers of Asthmatics (AANMA), the nonprofit clearing house and national learning center. Asthmatic herself and mother of asthmatic children, Nancy is a tireless advocate on the subject. What she says about asthma could easily be applied to your child's health with a little editing:

> "Take a moment to write a thank you letter to your airways for working so hard even when inflamed and

swollen. Thank the bronchial muscles wrapped around the airways for straining to keep the airways open despite mucous plugs and excess fluid oozing from ruptured cells lining the surface.

Let your mind reflect on all the many ways your airways serve you despite the abuse they take every time you go out with that handsome guy who smokes cigars. Appreciate the cilia lining the airways that sweep trapped dust, cat dander, and pollen-laden mucus particles up and out of the airways into your throat where you cough them up or swallow them down. Validate the mucus for trapping foreign invaders so they can't clog the air sacs and kill you.

Doing this exercise is more than therapeutic. It puts your mind in a receptive, appreciative, more powerful mode. When you learn about asthma, breathing, and your immune system, you stop thinking about the *disease* and start focusing on being good to your body. Suddenly, allergy-proofing the home isn't a chore or punishment; it's a healthier choice.

We can't change the fact that we have asthma, but we can change how we think about it and the way we treat ourselves. The more you know about asthma and treatment options, the more likely you'll make good choices and shorten the learning curve between where you are now and where you want to be."

What Nancy accomplishes very well in this extract is to show the body not as an enemy that has betrayed us somehow, but as a valiant ally that needs *our* help to do its work better, and the better the job we do of helping our bodies, the greater the payoff in our ability to enjoy life.

Over many years, we have seen time and time again in our practice that rather than allergy or asthma tethering a child and family to a limited existence, they can gain control over their life to a much greater extent and so widen the radius of activity.

Even in cases where peanut allergy, say, makes control a matter of life and death, the habits of mastering their environment can provide them with greater discipline and enjoyment of the aspects of their lives that are open to them. Once the debilitating effects of asthma are overcome, and the cycles of affliction and relief that come from too heavy reliance on rescue medication are broken, a great weight is often lifted. Instant gratification is not a part of the program. Knowledge, patience, and commitment are.

We allergists can only show you the way and give you the tools. But it is ultimately up to you, the parents, and your children to do the rest. By following the medication regimen, by cleaning up properly, by sacrificing certain aspects of your lifestyle, including sometimes a beloved pet, by eating right, by getting enough sleep, and so on. You will have help from the many parents and children nearby who have accomplished similar breakthroughs in their lives once you find them.

This is not a matter of luck. A very wise man, Branch Rickey, who ran a long-lost baseball team called the Brooklyn Dodgers, once said, "Luck is the residue of design." The design for better living is out there. Make it happen. But good luck anyway.

Treating Asthma in the Inner City, And What It Means For the Rest of the Country

B OTH OF US HAVE DEVOTED A CONSIDERABLE AMOUNT OF TIME TO disadvantaged urban populations in recent years. We realize that mainstream practice has its rewards, but the bigger pay-off, personally and for society as a whole, comes from extending our knowledge and experience to those who lack access to effective care.

The medical costs of untreated or undertreated chronic disease are well known, and are part of the current dialogue about health care reform. They increase exponentially as disease goes unmanaged. Contrary to what some politicians contend, emergency rooms do not provide health care.

But short of the emergency room, the costs can be counted in days lost at school and work (asthma is the number-one cause of absenteeism), diminished performance, inactivity, and poorer prospects for achievement through one's entire life. Nor are the bad effects confined to the individual child. As we have discussed in earlier, when one kid has uncontrolled asthma, the whole family gets sick. We realize we can't compensate for all the inequities that life deals these families, but where asthma is concerned, gains in quality of life and health for a single child can have exponential benefits for the child, the family, and the classroom. These are our testimonials:

America's Canary

O utside the window of the Urban Health clinic in the South Bronx where I work is a schoolyard. On a typical day, Hispanic and African American boys play basketball. After each basket, some players pause to use their asthma inhalers. As the game progresses, they get less and less relief. The Hispanic kids say they have *azma*.

In parts of the Bronx it is estimated that 20 percent of the children have asthma. Hospitalization rates for asthma in Bronx County and East Harlem are twenty-one times higher than those of affluent parts of the city. Hospitalization rates are 17.3 per 1,000 people and death rates 11 per 100,000, eight times the national average.

At Lincoln Hospital in the South Bronx, there are days when the special asthma room, where patients sit along a wall sucking on bronchial dilators, is chaotic as Lincoln doctors scramble to collect more information. Some patients are cocaine abusers, some are homeless, their medical records scattered at various clinics around the borough and effectively inaccessible.

This neighborhood, Hunts Point, is home to one of the largest wholesale produce markets in the nation, a large waste-disposal site, and multiple automobile junkyards. There are 10,000 workers in the area and 10,000 residents. Approximately one million trucks enter each year mostly late at night and in the early morning (as well as the traffic to nearby Yankee Stadium more than eighty times each season). Trucks wait in line to deliver their products while running their engines and exposing the environment to exhaust, both diesel and gasoline. Coal miners kept birds with them to warn of bad air building up. The South Bronx is America's canary because it points to what will happen in the rest of the country, if we allow air quality to deteriorate.

A generation ago, so many buildings were burnt to the ground that the police station, which remained standing, was known as Fort Apache. Today, community pride has rebuilt these neighborhoods, but bad air and asthma are part of the legacy.

In addition to vehicle-belched irritants, almost all area residents are affected by the allergens we have discussed throughout this book: indoor air pollution, in particular dust mites; cockroach feces and body parts; and rat and mouse urine.

The Bronx has more households with more than one person per room in the city: 16.6 percent compared with 12.3 percent citywide, which accelerates transmission of respiratory infections. Family stress is also seen as a factor.

I have had the privilege in recent years of working with the primary care physicians at Urban Health Plan. They were doing an excellent job in following NIH guidelines and caring for their primarily Hispanic asthmatics, when I came aboard to add specialty care. They had demonstrated a 30 percent savings for the average asthmatic compared to a major HMO.

My colleagues Dr. Acklema Mohammad and Sylvia Romero-Johnson, RN, developed the Asthma Relief Street Program, which takes an integrated approach in working with patients, their families, providers, and community agencies. A strong health education component reinforces self-management skills. Partnerships with community agencies integrate our work with that of other community agencies. Asthma Relief Street is available at all Urban Health Plan facilities, including five school-based health centers.

Patients have shown more symptom-free days, increased medication compliance, fewer urgent care and fewer emergency room visits, and better school attendance. (For information call Sylvia Romero-Johnson, asthma coordinator, 718-589-2440 ext. 4313.)

Another useful element is an emphasis on sleep medicine, which was introduced by Dr. Sam De Leon, a pulmonologist and sleep specialist, as well as chief medical officer. Snoring or obstructive sleep apnea can exacerbate asthma, diabetes, and many cardio-vascular conditions because of the stress they put on the heart and airways.

The primary care physicians at Urban Health Plan had done such a good job with the average asthmatic, what could we add with specialty care? Research by Regina Herzlinger of Harvard Business School shows that 20 percent of patients may account for 80 percent of the cost of treatment. So we made it a priority to identify the "worst of the worst" patients using the Plan's electronic medical records. These patients were assigned to me.

I feel very fortunate at this late date in my medical career to have a chance to work in this setting, with such dedicated, visionary doctors and other medical professionals. Our work will undoubtedly have utility in other urban as well as suburban and rural settings, where airborne pollution is also on the rise.

The South Bronx is a community of strivers, or potential strivers. The same businesses that they depend on are also, particularly in this concentration, the worst ones for their health. This is one place where a new, green transportation system would be a real boon.

You can see up close the treadmill that poverty represents. A $10-an-hour job disqualifies people from getting safety-net benefits, including Medicaid, so many who want to work can't afford to. Children may qualify for health insurance but their parents may not. Poor diets lead to obesity, high blood pressure, diabetes, sleep apnea and, of course, asthma; maybe we should call it poverty syndrome. We see homeless ex-cons who are placed in one shelter, and their families in another. This is hardly conducive to establishing the kind of routine needed to manage a chronic disease.

Then there is the resistance to mainstream medicine among Hispanic populations you read about in chapter 10. Their beliefs clash with what the doctor tells them. In the absence of overt symptoms, they prefer to use their accustomed medicines, such as whale oil and almond oil, to control their asthma, even though these can contain allergens themselves. The inflammation goes unchecked, until it boils over and they end up overusing their inhalers, or back in the emergency room.

Our obligation as physicians is clear: We must explain and demonstrate and monitor and explain again. We must gain trust.

— *Dr. Chiaramonte*

Specialists in the Schools

Early in 2005, a friend, Barbara Cutler, and I hatched a scheme to put asthma specialists in schools that had high concentrations of asthmatic children. Barbara, a lawyer by training, had long experience as New York's legal advocate for the city's homeless children.

Schools are the ideal setting for helping disadvantaged children with limited access to health care precisely because they are present regularly, which is especially important for a condition that requires systematic follow up. Working parents depend on their children's attendance at school to give them time to earn a living, and for the homeless, it provides one stable element in an often-chaotic existence.

Having the specialist in the school saves parents the burden of taking time off from work or finding care for their other children to go to a doctor who may be located across town. Even where asthma care is available in a community clinic, there is a high rate of attrition from treatment because of the inconvenience.

Schools are a useful base for asthma care for another reason. Teachers, administrators and, indeed, other students have a vested interest in keeping asthmatic children symptom free. Asthma is disruptive of the educational process for all these constituents as well as for patients.

We received sponsorship from Barbara's employer, the public relations firm Fleishman Hillard, for Project E.R.A.S.E, a pithy abbreviation for the ungainly name: Eradicating Respiratory Asthma in Schools to help children Excel. We also had support from the schools chancellor, Joel I. Klein.

In the fall of 2005, a colleague, Dr. Nathaniel Horne, and I began spending one morning a week at two New York City public elementary schools on the Lower East Side, meeting with a total of fifty-one children. Following physical examinations and securing medical histories supplied by the parents, the doctors worked with the children's primary care physicians, mostly at hospitals and clinics, on custom treatment plans. As doctors in private practice not employed by the Department of Education or the Department of Health, we were precluded by law from prescribing medication or performing invasive procedures, such as giving injections, in the schools, so we worked with their doctors.

We also worked regularly with the families on modifying behavior and hygiene in the home, with the aim of controlling inflammation and reducing exposure to allergens and other asthma triggers.

Care is provided at no cost to the students' families or to the school system.

Our objectives were to:

• Reduce asthma among the city's low-income minority children, beginning with targeted public schools in District 1
• Reduce asthma-related school absenteeism for these children
• Reduce asthma-related hospitalizations for this population
• Increase management skills among parents, caregivers, teachers, and children
• Create a model that can be replicated in other public school systems, regionally and nationally

The results were dramatic. Compared to the previous academic year: School absences fell by more than half (128 to 57); Emergency room visits fell by one-quarter (40 to 30); Hospitalizations fell by more than three-quarters (26 to 6).

In addition to the numerical results, feedback from the parents and school personnel showed that the program promoted greater understanding of the disease, reduced stress for patients and their families, improved both conduct and performance in the classroom, and increased participation in nonacademic activities. In one school, dedicated faculty started a running team, something previously unthinkable. They no longer disappeared into the background but wore their special T-shirts to school proudly. Parents eagerly received the information, made changes at home, and deeply appreciated their children's progress.

Even the prohibition on providing treatment directly to students had an unforeseen and highly beneficial side effect. Our partnership with doctors at clinics and even emergency rooms not only benefited asthma management, it extended a continuum of care that is not possible when patients visit a doctor only when they are symptomatic.

Project E.R.A.S.E. also made the doctors ourselves available by phone to patients and their families, as we are in private practice. This was a first for some families whose previous contact with doctors was largely under emergency conditions. We were similarly available to teachers and school administrators, anyone in a position to observe changes in the child's health and behavior that might indicate a problem with his or her asthma.

Leveraging our resources through primary care physicians and other channels in this way was in part the inspiration for creating AsthmaAllergiesChildren.com. Parents want information about their children and concerned physicians want access to new ideas for patients who don't respond to current treatment. Our website provides that.

In the years since, Project E.R.A.S.E. has added doctors and schools to our coverage, and received support from communities and politicians. It has also provided a foundation for further community outreach.

The upshot for me of this experience is that I see as never before how direct work with the neediest patients—the 20 percent Dr. Chiaramonte mentions above who cost 80 percent of the money— can make huge differences in their lives. That's why as time goes by I work very hard to persuade these patients to come to my office in Midtown Manhattan. There, I'm not bound by Department of Education rules, and I can use every sample and every bit of literature provided by Big Pharma to educate and treat patients and their families, at no cost to anyone.

These families don't "overuse" health care, a term flung around by ideologues who think consumer choice of how and where to spend health care dollars will reduce the nation's bills. Health care is not another consumer item, where patients of any socio-economic status can go to *Consumer Reports* and look for the "best buy."

No matter how the nation chooses to go forward with health care—whether reform becomes a reality, whether that reform is more than just a Band-aid, or whether we continue on the unsustainable path we're on—better management of chronic disease is a sure-fire winner. Today, whether the disease is asthma, diabetes, or obesity, that 20-80 rule applies. It doesn't have to be that way.

Specialty allergy and asthma care is already a best buy, and that is why I am already so involved in trying to promote it, even at my own expense, and looking for new ways to leverage what we know, which is why Larry and I have updated this book and built a website to go with it. My fondest hope is that this combination of print and electronics will have a fraction of the impact on the treatment of allergies and asthma at large that we see in our clinics day to day. Better breathing, better grades, better attendance at school and at work. Better lives.

— *Dr. Ehrlich*

Appendix:
Table of Medications

Allergic Rhinitis Medications

Generic Medication	Brand Name	OTC or Prescription	Age
diphenhydramine	Benadryl	OTC (over the counter)	6 months plus
chlorpheniramine	Chlor-Trimeton	OTC	12 years plus
loratadine	Claritin	OTC	2 months plus, depending on form
desloratadine	Clarinex	prescription	12 years plus
fexofenadine	Allegra	prescription	6 years plus
cetirizine	Zyrtec	OTC	1 year plus
levocetirizine	Xyzal	prescription	6 months plus
cromolyn sodium	NasalCrom	OTC	2 years plus
azelastine	Astepro 0.1% and 0.15%	prescription	5 years plus
montelukast	Singulair	prescription	2 years plus for allergic rhinitis (1 year plus for asthma)

Symptoms Treated	Side Effects (Most Common)	Special Notes
itching, watery nose, occasionally itching eyes	fatigue, dry mucous membranes	longest available antihistamine
itching, watery nose, occasionally itching eyes	fatigue, dry mucous membranes	none
itching, watery nose, occasionally itching eyes	fatigue, very rare	popular OTC medicine, few side effects
itching, watery nose, occasionally itching eyes & hives	occasional sore throat, dry mouth	long half life, decongests
nasal congestion, watery nose, itching due to eczema	occasional headache, upper respiratory infection	with and without pseudoephedrine (Sudafed)
nasal congestion, watery nose, itching due to eczema	sleepiness	with and without pseudoephedrine
nasal congestion, watery nose, itching due to eczema	occasional sleepiness	none
nasal congestion, watery nose	none	stabilizes mast cells
nasal congestion, watery nose	bloody nose	as antihistamine, may cause drowsiness
nasal congestion, watery nose	stomachache	may be used with all other allergic rhinitis drugs

Allergic Rhinitis Medications:
Intranasal Steroids (INS)*

Generic Medication	Brand Name	OTC or prescription	Age
budesonide*	Rhinocort Aqua	prescription	6 years plus*
fluticasone*	Flonase	prescription	4 years plus*
triamcinolone*	Nasacort AQ	prescription	6 years plus*
mometasone*	Nasonex	prescription	2 years plus*
beclomethasone*	Beconase	prescription	6 years plus*
fluticasone*	Veramyst	prescription	12 years plus*
ciclesonide*	Omnaris	prescription	6 years plus*

* The FDA recommends allowing INS in younger patients for short periods of time, as for seasonal allergic rhinitis.

Medications for Acute Allergic Reactions
(such as with food allergy)

Generic Medication	Brand Name	OTC or prescription	Age
epinephrine	Twinject, EpiPen	prescription	special smaller dosages available for children under 50 lbs.
diphenhydramine	Benadryl	OTC	6 months plus

Symptoms Treated	Side Effects (Most Common)	Special Notes
nasal congestion, watery nose	bloody nose	monitor child's growth
nasal congestion, watery nose	bloody nose	monitor child's growth
nasal congestion, watery nose	bloody nose	monitor child's growth
nasal congestion, watery nose	bloody nose	monitor child's growth
nasal congestion, watery nose	bloody nose, occasional sneezing attacks	monitor child's growth
nasal congestion, watery nose	bloody nose	monitor child's growth
nasal congestion, watery nose	bloody nose	monitor child's growth

Symptoms Treated	Side Effects (Most Common)	Special Notes
acute allergic reactions or anaphylaxis	rapid heart rate, high blood pressure	medical caregiver *must* instruct patient, parents, others how to use
acute allergic reactions or anaphylaxis	fatigue, dry mouth	effective OTC medication for all allergic reactions

Allergic Conjunctivitis Medications**

Generic Medication	Brand Name	OTC or prescription	Age
olopatadine hydrochloride	Patanol, Pataday	prescription	3 years plus
ketotifen	Zaditor	prescription	3 years plus
levocabastine	Livostin	prescription	12 years plus
azelastine hydrochloride	Optivar	prescription	3 years plus
antazoline + naphazoline	Vasocon-A	prescription	3 years plus
naphozoline + pheniramine maleate	Visine-A	prescription	consult doctor if under 6 years
nedocromil sodium	Alocril	prescription	3 years plus
lodoxamide	Alomide	OTC	3 years plus
ketorolac	Acular	OTC	3 years plus
bepotastine besilate	Bepreve	prescription	2 years plus

** All nonsteroidal: Never use steroids on eyes.

Symptoms Treated	Side Effects (Most Common)	Special Notes
itchy, watery eyes	headaches	inhibits release of histamine from mast cells
itchy eyes	headaches and rhinitis similar to allergies in general	antihistamine and mast cell stabilizer
itchy eyes	stinging and burning eyes	antihistamine
itchy eyes	stinging and burning eyes, bitter taste	antihistamine
itchy, red eyes	occasional burning eyes	ingestion by infants may produce coma
itchy, red eyes	pupils may become enlarged	consult doctor if eye pain or changes in visibility
itchy, tearing eyes	headaches, itchy or burning eyes	mast cell stabilizer
ocular inflammatory states such as vernal conjunctivitis, vernal keratitis, vernal keratoconjunctivitis	ocular discomfort, blurred vision, excessive tearing	mast cell stabilizer
itchy eyes due to seasonal conjunctivitis	bleeding, allergic reaction, rash	nonsteroidal anti-inflammatory drug (like aspirin)
itchy, watery eyes	slight taste	none

Asthma Medications

Generic Medication	Brand Name	OTC or prescription	Age
ephedrine	Primatene	OTC	6 years plus
theophylline	Theo-Dur, Slo-Bid, Uniphyl	prescription	6 months plus
montelukast	Singulair	prescription	2 years plus
zafirlukast	Accolate	prescription	5 years plus
albuterol	Ventolin, Proventil	prescription	1 year plus
pirbuterol	Maxair Autohaler	prescription	12 years plus
ipratropium	Atrovent	prescription	12 years plus

Symptoms Treated	Side Effects (Most Common)	Special Notes
bronchoconstriction only	central nervous system and cardiac stimulation, rise in blood pressure	*not recommended*
bronchoconstriction only	nausea	overdose may lead to convulsions or death; blood levels of theophylline must be measured
mild to severe asthma (used alone or in combination with other medications)	headache	not to be used for acute asthma attacks
mild to severe asthma (used alone or in combination with other medications)	headache	not to be used for acute asthma attacks
bronchoconstriction only	tremors, increased heart rates	reliever medication, for acute attacks only; should not be used as preventive; oral and nebulized medications must be used as doctor orders
bronchoconstriction only	tremors, increased heart rates (though less frequently than with albuterol)	metered-dose inhaler (MDI); breath-actuated, easy to use
bronchoconstriction only	headache, dizziness, dry mouth, nausea	*do not* use for acute asthma; do not use if soy-and/or peanut-allergic

Asthma Medications:
Long-Acting Beta-Agonists (LABAs)†

Generic Medication	Brand Name	OTC or prescription	Age
salmeterol†	Serevent	prescription	4 years plus
formoterol†	Foradil	prescription	5 years plus for chronic asthma; 12 years plus for exercise-induced asthma (EIA)

† The FDA recommends against using LABAs alone.

Asthma Medications:
Inhaled Corticosteroids (ICS)††

Generic Medication	Brand Name	OTC or prescription	Age
mometasone††	Asmanex	prescription	4 years plus
beclomethasone††	Qvar	prescription	5 years plus
budesonide††	Pulmicort	prescription	1 year plus
fluticasone††	Flovent	prescription	12 years plus

†† ICS should not be used for acute asthma. At high dosages, bone growth and pituitary gland function can be impaired, and thus should be monitored.

Symptoms Treated	Side Effects (Most Common)	Special Notes
bronchoconstriction only	see chapter 8 of this book; for updates, see asthmaallergieschildren. com	*do not use for acute asthma*[†]
bronchoconstriction only	rare tremors	FDA approved for daily use (chronic) and EIA[†]

Symptoms Treated	Side Effects (Most Common)	Special Notes
inflammation	[††]	[††]
inflammation	[††]	[††]
chronic asthmatic inflammation	[††]	may take weeks for maximum effect; can be used with Foradil
chronic asthmatic inflammation	[††]	can be used with Foradil; comes in three concentrations

Asthma Medications: Combined LABA and ICS

Generic Medication	Brand Name	OTC or prescription	Age
fluticasone / salmeterol	Advair	prescription	12 years plus
formoterol / budesonide	Symbicort	prescription	12 years plus (soon to be lowered)

Leading-Edge Asthma Medication

Generic Medication	Brand Name	OTC or prescription	Age
anti-IgE antibody	Xolair	prescription	12 years plus

Symptoms Treated	Side Effects (Most Common)	Special Notes
bronchoconstriction, inflammation	increased heart rate, tremors, oral candida infections	growth and pituitary gland should be monitored; comes in three concentrations
bronchoconstriction, inflammation	increased heart rate, tremors, oral candida infections	growth and pituitary gland should be monitored

Symptoms Treated	Side Effects (Most Common)	Special Notes
severe persistent asthma, inflammation	occasional allergic reactions	high cost limits use; injectable only; used with steroids

Index

About the Authors

DR. PAUL M. EHRLICH WAS EDUCATED AT COLUMBIA UNIVERSITY AND studied medicine at New York University School of Medicine. He trained in pediatrics at Bellevue Hospital at NYU, and allergy and immunology at Walter Reed Army Medical Center. He is a partner at Allergy and Asthma Associates of Murray Hill, clinical assistant professor of pediatrics at New York University School of Medicine, attending physician in medicine and pediatrics at Beth Israel Medical Center, and attending physician at the New York Eye & Ear Infirmary, all in New York City.

Dr. Ehrlich is a fellow of the American Academy of Pediatrics, the American Academy of Allergy, Asthma & Immunology, and the American College of Allergy, Asthma & Immunology. He has been featured as one the top pediatric allergy and immunology specialists in *New York Magazine* for the last nine years and counting.

DR. LARRY CHIARAMONTE WAS EDUCATED AT YALE COLLEGE and trained in family practice, pediatrics, and allergy and immunology at Yale and John Hopkins. He has done groundbreaking research as well as clinical practice. He established a program that produced dozens of allergists in Brooklyn, New York, with a focus on inner-city populations. His work on compliance and use of peak flow meters are now part of the national guidelines for the treatment of allergy. He also started the first food allergy center in New York City and has undertaken several surveys with the NPI group regarding American's beliefs about food allergy.

Dr. Chiaramonte is now concentrating on asthma treatment relating to Ground Zero in Lower Manhattan and in high-risk populations in the South Bronx.

CPSIA information can be obtained at www.ICGtesting.com
Printed in the USA
BVOW04s1801210115

384282BV00011B/284/P